Contents

Preface to the seventh edition

Welcome! Twenty years ago, Peter wrote the first edition of this guide to help improve doctors' communication skills. Since then much in medicine has progressed but people have not. They still get confused and frightened by illness and treatments, and doctors still tend to forget this. Our patients are changed in some important ways, though; they are both blessed and cursed by the explosion of Internet knowledge.

Peter's father was a doctor in South Shields, on the Tyne. He qualified in 1938, and he knew a lot more about health and illness than his patients. He was wrong about a lot of stuff, as was the medical profession generally, but he was seen as a fount of knowledge and later as a repository of experiential wisdom. Peter qualified in 1968, and at the beginning of his career was perceived in a similar way to his father by those patients who came into contact with him. He was also wrong about a lot of stuff. He thought duodenal ulcers were caused by smoking and were best treated by putting sufferers in hospital and drip feeding them milk directly into their stomachs – and there was much else that was gospel at the time but is now considered silly. However, despite this, he was also seen as a medical repository of knowledge, and even his junior doctor word was taken as holy writ by most of his patients. This is not going to happen to you, and you know it.

Access to information has changed fundamentally, and this is changing communication between healthcare professionals and their patients. The man or woman in the street, on the bus or in the outpatients department can now unlock almost unlimited medical knowledge with minimal effort, and if the circumstances of their lives dictate it, they will seek this information out.

This fundamentally changes the expectations that you might have had about your role as a doctor. Previous generations doled out knowledge to patients in carefully titrated doses, but withheld enough information to retain power of influence. You cannot do that.

In 2014–15, as soon as an individual or a member of their family experiences a major health event, someone in that circle will seek out information, usually by means of a few swipes of a smartphone or clicks of a mouse button. Within minutes they will have more information on the subject than you can possibly carry in your head. This is a huge change for doctors. Since recorded history, and from anthropological research even before that, doctors, shamans and priests have controlled medical knowledge. However, the genie is now out of the bottle, and he demands a different form of communication to that to which medics have become accustomed for thousands of years. This recent, monumental shift demands a different approach, so to help you negotiate the changing world Peter and his daughter Liz have teamed up to pool their experience.

Liz is an NHS psychiatrist who qualified from Southampton Medical School in 2004 and has travelled those oh-so-difficult first years much more recently than her increasingly dated but battle-hardened parent. Her experience of working and training in the modern NHS, and now educating the next generation of trainees in communication, ensures this latest edition is current and relevant to all of you. This also heralds a change in emphasis from being a guide essentially for young GPs to a handbook for all young (and not so young) doctors in whatever speciality.

We hope to help you to make this epoch-changing transition from teller and controller to listener, sharer and interpreter. In this seventh edition we have tried to do more than just update things – we want to help you get ahead of the pack, to really enjoy your job and to gain increased professional satisfaction from communicating effectively with your patients. We will argue that doctors are even more important than before. Ironically, with so much information around, patients are often very confused and even more anxious. Influencing patient health is not all about prescribing drugs and we must recognise the value of communication as a core therapeutic intervention rather than just a nice thing to do or a way to pass exams. Many more allied healthcare professionals are now taking on roles that were traditionally medical, and patients are much better informed, so what is it about us that is still unique and valuable? If you don't know already, this little book will soon remind you that there is ample evidence that the majority of patients don't take the treatments we prescribe them anyway. We need to do better, and psychologically informed communication is essential. It is a stark fact that most complaints about us are related to failures of communication rather than poor clinical skills.

Since the first edition there have been major changes to acceptable ethics of clinical practice. For example, it used to be considered detrimental to disclose bad news to patients, especially in hospital practice. Until very recently many doctors were still covertly medicating patients, but changes in mental capacity and mental health law have now effectively outlawed this practice. Openness, honesty and transparency are the order of the day, along with patient autonomy, and this can be tricky for those of us not prepared for this approach.

Finally, we must admit to ourselves that the biggest determinants of health are often social not medical – employment being one of the biggest, which means understanding about the whole person *is* medical treatment. Virchow said *medicine is a social science and politics is just medicine on a larger scale.*

Good reading.

Peter and Liz Tate
March 2014
peter.spud@gmail.com
liztate@doctors.org.uk

About the authors

Peter Tate

Peter Tate was 21 when he qualified in 1968. After spells as a P&O surgeon and as a trainee in Kentish Town he was a GP in Abingdon for 30 years. He was a GP trainer for 25 years, an MRCGP examiner from 1981, retiring as convenor of the panel of examiners in March 2006. He wrote the first edition of *The Doctor's Communication Handbook* in 1993. The book won the leading French medical literary prize, Prix Prescire, in October 2006 and has been translated into six languages. He is also the author of *The Other Side of Medicine*, a collection of essays and short stories and co-author of *The Consultation* and *The New Consultation* (both published by Oxford University Press). In the last couple of years he has written and presented three educational DVDs for doctors. He was awarded the MBE in 2008 and was jointly awarded the prestigious Lynn Payer Award for outstanding contributions to the literature of the teaching of effective healthcare communication by the American Academy on Communication in Healthcare (AACH) in October 2011. (See: www.thetates.me/)

Liz Tate

Liz Tate qualified from Southampton in 2004 after completing an intercalated degree. She did her pre-registration year in Southampton General and still wakes up in a cold sweat on occasion when remembering weeks of nights as a very inexperienced doctor responsible for what seemed like hundreds of very sick patients spread all over the hospital. She then undertook placements in medicine, palliative care and psychiatry. Much to her surprise she loved the psychiatry job the most and was subsequently accepted onto the Wessex Psychiatry Rotation. She felt the full force of MTAS and for a while a move to

Australia was on the cards, but she was one of the lucky ones who was eventually reappointed to the same job and continued training in Wessex. She specialises in forensic psychiatry, which involves looking after some of the most complex and challenging patients in medicine.

Having dabbled in teaching since medical school, in 2012 she was awarded a fellowship in education to design a new training programme for psychiatry trainees in Wessex. She has gone on to develop new modules for the MRCPsych course, and teaches facilitation and communication skills on behalf of Wessex Deanery. She was appointed a Medical Education Fellow in Wessex in 2014.

What I bring to the party

The Doctor's Communication Handbook has been an established and respected brand for nearly 20 years. The first edition was published long before I even started medical school and over the years has evolved to incorporate a lifetime of experience and research. During medical school I lost count of the number of times people waxed lyrical about it to me, only to be dumbstruck when they realised the connection. It was something of a surprise to me when I finally read it and began to realise why people were so passionate about it. I never imagined that 15 years on I would be contributing to the seventh edition!

For me the unique selling point of the handbook is the friendly style and personal narrative which people have often said makes them feel like they are talking to a helpful and sympathetic colleague rather than reading a textbook. I hope we have enhanced this style in the latest edition and maintained the family feel by literally adding another family member!

Liz Tate
March 2014

CHAPTER 1

Ideas, concerns and expectations

The White Rabbit put on his spectacles.
'Where shall I begin, please your Majesty?'
'Begin at the beginning,' the King said gravely, 'and go on till
you come to the end: then stop.'

Alice's Adventures in Wonderland, 1865

Some early truths to remember

For those of you at the beginning of your journey, here are some fundamental truths to remember. For those of you further down the path, take a minute to remind yourself of these and think about how often you take them into account when you talk to your patients.

- The patient is a lot more frightened than you are.
- The patient thinks it is more serious than you do.
- Illness is frightening, but understanding what is going on helps. This applies both to the patient and to you.
- Taking a history is a method of controlling what the patient says.

This book is a guide to help you talk with, understand and share with your patients. It will not teach you the traditional medical history-taking model, but it may help you to use that model more effectively both for yourself and for your patients.

Those first encounters with real people who have come to you for help in the hospital or the outpatients department are very daunting. We all suffer the anxiety of being found wanting, of getting it wrong, of being harshly criticised by our teachers or, worst of all, just looking foolish. *The best way to start is to think ourselves into the role of patient.* After all, this is not too difficult – we have all been ill at some time and we all shall be again. When people become ill they ask themselves several questions, such as 'What has happened?', 'Why has it happened?', 'Why has it happened to me?', 'Why now?', 'What should I do about it?', 'Should I go to the doctor?', 'Is it serious?' and 'Can it be treated?' Think of the last patient you saw. What questions do you think they had asked themselves? Imagine that that patient was you. What would you be asking yourself?

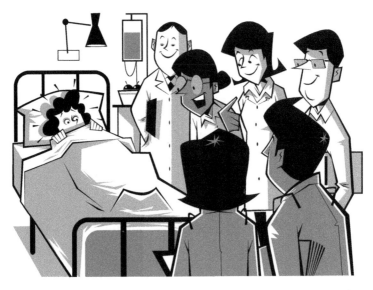

Let us suppose that the last patient you saw was in surgical outpatients and she was a 35-year-old woman presenting to the clinic with a nodular goitre. You have taken her history and found out that she is married with no children. She first noticed a swelling in her neck about six months ago, she went to her GP three months ago, and she has waited for the outpatient appointment since her second visit to the GP two and a half months ago. The GP has stated in his letter that the thyroid function tests were borderline normal and that there is no family history of thyroid disease. In your detailed and systematic history taking you have not discovered any symptoms referable to the thyroid gland, but the patient does seem to be rather anxious. Examination confirms a moderately enlarged gland with multiple small nodules, everything else is normal, but the patient seems to be slightly trembly and perhaps sweating more than you would expect. Now step aside from your history and examination and ask yourself what she might be thinking and feeling. Now do it again.

Let us just consider some of her possible thoughts and feelings. First, she is certainly frightened. Hospitals are terrifying places to most people – they are pain and death boxes with a funny smell. She is also afraid of the staff, especially the doctors, *including you*. Doctors are frightening for several reasons, not least their association with the mysteries of life and death. They also tend to be dominant, powerful figures who have control over one's immediate and even long-term future. This patient knows that many doctors do not say very much, and what they do say can be difficult to understand. She also knows that doctors usually do not tell the whole truth.

She is also very concerned about herself. She has a lumpy enlargement in her neck, which to her is cancer until proved otherwise, and she will take a lot of convincing because her aunt died of cancer of the gullet (oesophagus to you) and she had lumps in her neck. She remembers that her aunt's doctors lied to her aunt, and that the treatment was horrible and ineffective. She has vaguely heard about the thyroid gland, and knows from a friend that one of the treatments is radioactive. This concerns her because she desperately wants children, she knows time is passing and she fears that a dose of radioactivity may put paid to her chances forever. She is also afraid of having an operation because she has never been in hospital and hates the idea of being 'put to sleep'. She does not wish to lose control. She also knows from friends, television and everyday experiences that operations can go wrong, and the neck seems to be a pretty dodgy place. Her husband produced a bundle of printouts from three websites he had found on the Internet about the thyroid gland. She did not understand much of this information, and could not bring herself to read some of the more alarming bits. She wishes that her husband was with her, but worries that he has not really wanted to talk about her neck or her coming to the hospital. She wonders if she is now ugly and unattractive. The bottom line is that she does not want to die.

The above description is only an imaginative guess at some of our patient's feelings, but how much of this did your history reveal, do you think? Is it important to know? Hopefully, your answer is yes, but not everyone would agree. Liz was somewhat surprised recently to encounter a psychiatry trainee who trained as a GP in Europe. He was adamant that the role of the doctor was to diagnose and treat illness, and that understanding the patient's thoughts and feelings on the matter was entirely separate and, to his way of thinking, unimportant.

Imagine you recite the findings of your history and examination to your chief. She listens and asks both you and your patient (let us call her Mrs Arthur) a few clarifying questions, and examines the thyroid gland herself. She excuses herself to Mrs Arthur and discusses the options with you while the patient listens.

Dr: Multinodular goitre is a difficult clinical area. Probably the best treatment is nothing if the patient can accept the cosmetic deformity. Some centres use thyroxine replacement, but you only get regression in 10%–20% of cases. The real patient worry is cancer, isn't that so, Mrs Arthur?

Mrs A, a little startled, nods in agreement.

Dr: Cancer isn't really a problem. The Framingham Study didn't find any in a 15-year follow-up of this sort of goitre, but it remains a theoretical risk, and if you give enough of any thyroid gland to a pathologist he will find some sort of cancer. We will scan it anyway. (*See* cautionary reference below.[*])

The real problem we have here with Mrs Arthur is of possible toxicity and the best treatment. The GP's thyroid function tests were borderline high, and Mrs Arthur's clinical state is possibly a little suggestive of hyperactivity. We should repeat the tests and

---

* Before continuing, we should mention that this example was used in the first edition of this book in 1994. This is the recommendation of the *British Medical Journal* article on the subject (Brito *et al.*, 2013):

> Uncertainty about the benefits and harms of immediate treatment for low risk papillary thyroid carcinoma should spur clinicians to engage patients in shared decision making. This will ensure treatment is consistent with the evidence for the subtype of cancer that they have and with their preferences. Some patients may prefer not to have aggressive treatment of small, low risk thyroid cancers, especially those patients where the risk clearly outweighs the benefits of treatment (for example, older patients, patients with other malignancies, or patients with severe comorbidities). Patients can be reassured that if nodules later show more aggressive behaviour the evidence suggests no additional harm from delayed surgical treatment.

if they are quite high give her treatment with radioactive iodine. If
that is not successful the next step would be an operation.
Dr [smiles at Mrs Arthur and leaves the room, saying]: The student
will explain it all to you. Don't worry, you are in good hands.

How well do you think you would handle this? What would you say
about the scan? What do you think the patient's feelings would be
on her way home? What might she say to her husband? Would she
come back for the ^{131}I treatment? How helpful was your history in
this context?

Mrs Arthur will appear again later on, so keep her in mind.
Now think about the last time you were ill. If you are always healthy,

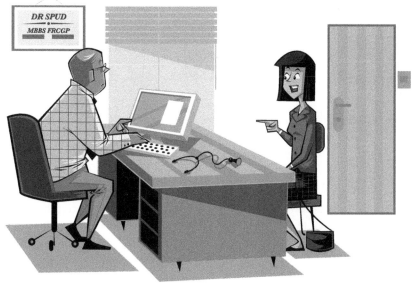

" I AM SORRY MRS ARTHUR BUT YOU DON'T UNDERSTAND."
" NO DOCTOR, I AM SORRY BUT YOU DON'T UNDERSTAND! "

take a moment to get into role and imagine waking with a severe sore
throat with a lot of swollen neck glands and feeling pretty ropey. Do
you go to the doctor? If so, why? If not, why not? What did you tell
yourself was happening? What was your worst case scenario? Did
you/would you have anyone to confide in? Did you/would you share
your fears? What questions would you ask yourself?

Let us go through some of your possible questions and answers:

1 *What has happened?* It's probably just a virus – Max had it last week.
2 *Why has it happened?* I've been working late, a bit overtired, resistance a bit low.
3 *Why has it happened to me?* Rotten luck, but I always get these things – Max sneezed over me.
4 *What should I do about it?* Dose myself up with soluble aspirin and it should just go.
5 *Is it serious?* No, it will be gone in a few days.

But what happens if your exams are two weeks away or you have a trip to the USA planned for next week?

1 *What has happened?* Oh no, maybe it is a streptococcus. I can't be ill now.
2 *What should I do about it?* I'd better get some antibiotics just in case. Maybe take some time off to nip it in the bud. Perhaps some vitamin C might help?
3 *Is it serious?* This might make me fail my exam. This will ruin my trip.

Now imagine that your partner has glandular fever.

1 *What has happened?* Oh God, it's glandular fever.
2 *Why has it happened?* It's Max's fault for kissing me.
3 *Why has it happened to me?* I had it coming – life has been too good recently.
4 *What should I do about it?* I'd better see the doc and get the test done to prove it.
5 *Is it serious?* Yes, this could put me out for the rest of the year. I've also read that it can cause Hodgkin's disease – oh my God!

These questions and answers can be translated into the trinity of *ideas*, *concerns* and *expectations*. To continue with the sore throat and glands scenario, consider what *ideas* might be going through your head that first morning:

I feel awful. Really, really bad. Too bad for a cold. It must be flu at the very least. I bet I got it from Max. He was coughing and sneezing all over me last week. It might be streptococcal, so a trip to the GP for some penicillin might help. I wonder if there is any on the ward I could have. I shall have to get some soluble aspirin.

What *concerns* might be running through your mind?

Help, I hope and pray it's not glandular fever. If it is, that's the exams down the tubes, and it can lead to Hodgkin's, can't it? What if it's worse? I mean acute leukaemia can start like this. I have been worrying about my immune system for some time. I haven't caught HIV from that needlestick in the Emergency Department, have I? No, that's silly, but it could turn into quinsy like that poor bloke on the ENT ward last week. His tonsils were so big he couldn't breathe. If I don't get this fixed pretty quickly, next week's trip to the USA is finito.

What about your *expectations*?

If I do nothing except dose myself up it will probably go away, but penicillin is a good idea because it might speed things up, especially with the USA trip coming up. I expect the old GP will just tell me it's a virus and I will have to lay it on a bit thick to get the penicillin. He might do a blood test for glandular fever. Shall I tell him I'm a bit worried about HIV? No, he will think I'm being silly. I expect he will tell me off for smoking, too.

Now think about Mrs Arthur again, and consider what sorts of things were going through her mind before she went to her GP for the first time. What she did *not* do was go to him with a nodular goitre. She went because she had certain ideas about the lumpy swelling in her neck. She had several concerns and a few hazy expectations.

Nobody goes to a doctor with just a symptom. They go with **ideas** about the symptom, with **concerns** about the symptom and with **expectations** related to the symptom.

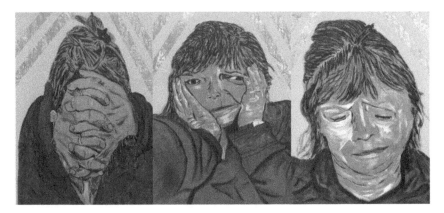

Triptych: ideas, concerns and expectations. By PT (mixed media)

Reference

Brito JP, Morris JC, Montori VM. Thyroid cancer: zealous imaging has increased detection and treatment of low risk tumours. *BMJ*. 2013; **347**: f4706.

CHAPTER 2

How doctors talk to patients and why

The two words 'information' and 'communication' are often used interchangeably, but they signify quite different things. Information is giving out; communication is getting through.

Sydney J Harris

- Asking questions only gets you answers.
- It is not whether the communication between doctor and patient is good or bad that matters, it is whether it is more or less *effective*.

For over 5000 years now the basic style of doctoring can be described in the modern ethical jargon as beneficent paternalism. The medical profession has thus adopted a well-meaning parental role in most patient encounters. Doctors have acted on behalf of, and for the good of, their patients. They have also wielded power over them. This role, which is taken for granted by our society, produces recognisable patterns of behaviour, which are disease-orientated with a strong tendency towards authoritarianism. It has become clear in recent years that this behaviour affords the doctor some emotional protection – in fact often more perceived than real – and is one of the most important reasons why many doctors find a more sharing approach so difficult.

Agendas

One way to think about the ways in which doctors communicate is to consider the *agendas* for both doctor and patient. Figure 2.1 demonstrates diagrammatically the possible spectrum of doctor communication behaviour with patients.

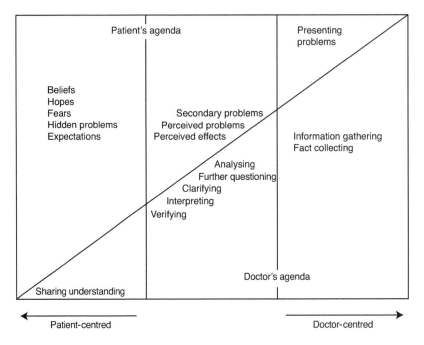

FIGURE 2.1 A power-shift model of styles of consultation

The right-hand side of the graph is nearly all doctor's agenda, with only the presenting complaint coming from the patient. As the doctor's style moves to the left, more and more of the patient's agenda is taken on board, until at the left-hand end of the graph it is nearly all patient's agenda. Most hospital doctors and still the majority of GPs tend towards the right-hand end of this model. This is not too surprising, as it is the way we are taught and for UK GPs, frighteningly, the way they are paid.

The whole act of *taking* a history is doctor-centred, and it is not necessarily bad in itself. Medical thoroughness and good pattern recognition are a hallmark of this style when practised well.

As an example of doctor-centred behaviour, imagine Mrs Arthur's first outpatient appointment. It could go something like this:

> Dr: Good morning, Mrs Arthur. Your GP says you seem to have a problem with your thyroid gland. Tell me, have you lost weight?
> Mrs A: No.
> Dr: Any hot flushes?
> Mrs A: No.
> Dr: Feeling tired or slowed up?
> Mrs A: Er, well, maybe a little, doctor.
> Dr: Bowels OK? Not constipated are you?
> Mrs A: Not really, doctor, I was wondering . . .
> Dr: I think I should examine you now. Would you take your blouse off . . .?

Mrs Arthur's agenda has not figured in the conversation so far – only the doctor's agenda is being addressed. Our European friend mentioned in Chapter 1 would be much happier if there was an effective test for every medical condition, negating the need to talk to patients at all.

Here is an example of a more patient-centred style, using the same scenario:

> Dr: Good morning, Mrs Arthur. Your GP says you have a problem with your thyroid gland. Would you tell me about it?
> Mrs A: Oh, er, well yes, I first noticed the swelling a few months ago, but I didn't do anything about it for a while.
> Dr: Why not?
> Mrs A: Oh, you know, I hoped it would go away while fearing the worst.
> Dr: The worst?
> Mrs A: Cancer, what else?
> Dr: That's a frightening thought. Do you still think it may be cancer?
> Mrs A: Well, yes, but I'm hoping you will be able to tell me, doctor.

In this example the patient's agenda figures highly to start with, and the doctor has not yet started on his agenda.

The totally patient-centred doctor is probably a dangerous creature. Patients do after all come for medical advice and considered professional opinions. They don't generally expect doctors to let them do all the talking, planning and managing (although in some cases this may be appropriate). One very intelligent, well-informed patient was nonetheless somewhat disconcerted, and not hugely reassured, when during a review of his anti-acid medication following a duodenal ulcer, his GP put their feet on the table and threw the BNF at him, saying, 'Choose whatever you like.'

However, the first chapter may have got you thinking that the doctor should, more often than not, take on board some of the patient's belief systems. An ideal doctor might perhaps lie around the middle of this spectrum, changing their behaviour one way or the other depending on the needs of the patient and the situation.

The problem as shown by experience and research is that doctors *do not change*. Audio and visual recordings of multiple consultations by the same doctor show a remarkable consistency of style. A simple analogy likens us to the traditional Englishman abroad. We don't act differently – we just talk more loudly or slowly. Thus doctors say and do things in much the same way with an anxious 16-year-old coming for a termination as with a 50-year-old woman with menorrhagia or an 80-year-old woman with vulval carcinoma. It appears that we do not regularly adapt to meet the needs of the patient. You could say that this does not matter so long as we have an effective set of behaviours with which we can cope with most patients. However, Chapter 3 will demonstrate that different patients need different types of communication. We need to be flexible, and it appears that most us of are not.

The most basic communication need is to discover why our patient has come to see us. This seems almost too obvious to state, but much research work suggests that doctors are not very good at it. In many consultations, doctors and patients do not appear to be talking about the same thing. Many years ago one of the truly great academic GPs, Professor Pat Byrne, gave this type of communication the deliberately ugly name of *dysfunctional*. In this sort of consultation the doctor and the patient are each pursuing their own quite separate agendas.

Doctors are good at diagnosis (i.e. establishing in the medical sense why a patient has come to see them). We discover the nature and history of the problem and the likely cause, but we tend not to be good at searching out our patients' beliefs and expectations. These are the real reasons why patients come to see us, and not discovering them can lead to a mismatch of agendas.

For example, a gloomy 64-year-old man comes to his GP for a sick note. The doctor knows this person to be a somewhat aggressive, paranoid and depressed individual with a long history of repeated admissions to a psychiatric hospital. The man says that he has been in hospital recently, and asks for a certificate. The doctor, seeing no record of the latest admission, but assuming that the usual has occurred, acquiesces quickly. He wants to avoid any difficult confrontation, and therefore fills in a certificate stating 'depression'. The doctor and patient briefly discuss convalescence and returning to work, and the patient leaves.

What is wrong with this scenario? Almost everything! The whole consultation was based on a false premise. The patient had in fact been admitted to hospital with a myocardial infarction. The doctor's original assumption was false, and nothing in the ensuing communication put it right. The doctor had failed to discover why his patient was there, and the patient did not realise this.

Dysfunctional communication is common in general practice because the patient's reason for coming to see their doctor is often unclear, but major misunderstandings do occur regularly in hospital. Consider the case of Mrs Arthur again. Let us carry on with the doctor-centred example given earlier in this chapter. Assume that the doctor has examined Mrs Arthur and completed the history taking in the form of a series of staccato questions. Mrs Arthur has therefore contributed none of her own thoughts and feelings. The time for explanation and management has come:

> Dr: Well, Mrs Arthur, there is nothing to worry about. You have multi-nodular goitre, but this is a benign condition. There are a couple more tests we need to do just to be on the safe side. I will arrange for a special scan and a biopsy of that biggish lump. Is that OK?
>
> Mrs A: So you are sure it is not serious, doctor?
>
> Dr: Oh yes. Speak to the nurse about the arrangements for the tests and I will see you in a month. Goodbye.
>
> Mrs A: Well, goodbye doctor, er, thank you.

This is deficient communication. The patient has not had any of her agenda addressed. Consider her ideas in Chapter 1. She has not been reassured about her future. She will probably attend for the tests out of fear, but she may default. She is not sure what the words 'multi-nodular', 'goitre', 'benign', 'special scan' or 'biopsy' mean, and she will go home feeling frustrated and afraid. The doctor, in turn, has focused his attention on the thyroid gland to the exclusion of everything else. He knows little about Mrs Arthur and nothing about her specific fears or reasons for consulting. This encounter is truly dysfunctional.

Power

Look at Figure 2.1 again and think about *power*. This type of diagram is known as a power-shift model. The doctor is much more in control on the right-hand side, and his power slips away as the agenda increasingly becomes that of the patient. This is not to say that the totally patient-centred doctor does not have power. They simply have less direct control and are much less authoritarian. It is worth stopping here to consider the nature of doctor power.

Patients expect and often want a powerful doctor; that is, a doctor who has reassuring authority, who is apparently capable and whose pronouncements can reduce anxiety. One definition of medical or 'Aesculapean' authority divides it into three parts – *sapiental, moral* and *charismatic*. These words are somewhat off-putting at first meeting, but bear with us.

Sapiential authority

This can be defined as the right to be heard, based on knowledge or expertise, and it means that doctors must know, or at least appear to know, more about medicine than their patients. However, this can only be one part of the doctor's authority, as a biochemist may know more about a particular branch of medicine, but it is to a physician that a patient turns when they are in need. Moreover, as we discussed at the beginning of the book, this knowledge is now much more freely available, thus reducing the intrinsic sapiential power of modern doctors.

Moral authority

This is the right to control and direct patients significantly, based on doing what society expects of us as doctors. In order to retain their moral authority, doctors must always act with the good of the patient as their paramount concern. This is derived from the Hippocratic credo. In addition, societies generally revere doctors, which means that doctors' behaviour is seen as socially right, as well as individually good. This is a powerful combination.

It is important to remember that it is not our role to be the purveyors of moral authority. We must remain impartial and avoid doing too much intrusive behaviour changing despite the pressures and expectations of government.

Charismatic authority

This is the most difficult of the three concepts, and it is similar to the anthropological definition of magic. It stems from the original unity between medicine and religion. In Western culture it is related to the possibility of death, and the magnitude of the issues with which the doctor deals. Many patients want doctors to be a little magical. For most of us when we are ill there is a need to supplement sapiential and moral authority with an ineffable factor, which might just hold out hope against the odds. Some doctors, particularly in the private sector, go out of their way to cultivate this. They develop a priestly mien, use complicated and obscure rituals, and act more like bishops than physicians.

The three forms of authority are present in all doctors, although some doctors go out of their way to develop particular sapiential, moral and charismatic elements in their behaviour towards patients and others. Think about some of the powerful doctors you have met and the nature of their power.

Here is an example. A partially patient-centred doctor, like that shown in Figure 2.1, has the same moral authority as their doctor-centred colleague, but they may reduce some of their sapiential authority by sharing more information with their patients. This highlights a fundamental truth. *Controlling information increases doctor power and restricts patient involvement.* Many doctors still become very uneasy with knowledgeable and inquisitive patients, as such patients decrease the doctor's control. The partially patient-centred doctor will also be more likely to attempt to demystify the nature of medical diagnosis and treatment, reducing their charismatic authority and thus their power to control the interview. This requires a degree of bravery, particularly when first trying such strategies.

Many doctors are afraid of losing this control – of exposing too much of their patient's pain and fear. You may find yourself not asking the important question due to a fear of opening an emotional Pandora's box and becoming overwhelmed. Such doctors use their power over their patient to keep the box shut and emotions at a non-threatening level. This style of behaviour can then become fixed and persist throughout a career. Don't let this happen to you, or you will lose much more than you gain. Inevitably, the fear of losing control of the interaction is most acute as a relatively junior doctor. This is the time of your life when the need to appear to know more than your patient can easily make you appear dismissive and unempathetic. Can we reassure you now that admitting knowledge gaps is not the end of your authority? It may be the beginning of a truly therapeutic relationship.

Doctors can increase their charismatic power, should they wish to do so, in many different ways. The trappings of power are the most obvious; for example, white coats, impressive mysterious gadgetry, attached (subservient) staff, a large desk with a big chair placed firmly behind it, grandiose-looking certificates on the wall, and computers with unintelligible displays or pointing away from the patient. Such doctors may communicate by means of cryptic oracle-like pronouncements, shrouded in 'medico-speak'. This can then be wrapped up with dire warnings of the fearsome consequences of not following the treatment properly, in order to complete the effect. Powerful rituals such as examining and prescribing are more charismatic in the absence of adequate explanations.

The problem with this contrived exercising of medical authority is that the overwhelming evidence suggests that *it is not very effective*. It quite obviously does not increase patient understanding, because that is not what is motivating the doctor. The often quoted reason for this style of communication is that it will make patients do what is good for them. However, the sad fact of the matter seems to be that more often than not they don't. The literature on adherence with medical advice reflects rather badly on doctors.

The *rule of one-thirds* describes this. It is easy to remember and is well authenticated:

- One-third of patients take medical advice and act in accordance with it sufficient for the advice to be effective.
- One-third take heed of some of the advice, but not enough for it to be effective. Imagine the way that many doctors take pills for a sore throat – a few one day when it is sore, forget for a day or so, and then start again when the throat gets sore again.
- One-third just don't bother.

For the seventh edition of this handbook it would be encouraging to report that recent evidence has shown this trend to be improving. Sadly, this is still not so. In many cases, especially in psychiatry, the rule of one-thirds appears to err greatly on the optimistic side.

Take the common life-threatening condition of type 2 diabetes, an illness that leads to blindness, terrible circulatory problems and considerable morbidity. Many patients need at least two drugs to control their blood-sugar level adequately. The modern rash of protocols usually assumes 100% adherence to prescribing regimes. So what are the facts? In a careful and thorough study of 1000 diabetic patients from Tayside in Scotland, reported in early 2000, the authors showed that adherence to a one-drug regime did indeed fit with the rule of one-thirds, with 33% of patients taking the medication as prescribed. However, when two drugs were prescribed the adherence fell to 13%! A review of the literature in 2005 revealed that long-term adherence to drug treatment decreased over time, and that 50% was an average figure after 3 years. There is an excellent review of this complex field in an open-access article in *Patient Preference and Adherence* (Blackburn *et al.*, 2013).

Think about this long and hard. You want to be the finest doctor in the land – to be able to recognise a yellow nail syndrome at 20 feet, to restore ailing people to full vigour with your hard-earned expertise – but in some cases more than two-thirds of your patients don't follow your advice. If your patients are really like that, how much use are you? How can you make sure that this fate won't befall you? Do you have to be in absolute control? (You already know the answer to this!)

In 2014 the term 'compliance' with therapy, which implies a subservient relationship, is still commonly used, particularly in the context of us pronouncing patients 'non-compliant'. Some still advocate the use of the term *'concordance'* instead, defined as a negotiated, shared agreement between clinician and patient concerning treatment regimen(s), outcomes, and behaviours; a more cooperative relationship than those based on issues of compliance, non-compliance and adherence, and we share this view. Most academics now prefer 'adherence' which even has its own cumbersome WHO definition. What is clear is that the slavish following of medical advice by patients is not only an unusual behaviour, but appears to be so uncommon in many cases as to be regarded as deviant.

Now think about this. We repeat that you are living through a time of historic change in the role of doctors. You are no longer the keeper of occult secrets, you are not the fount of all medical wisdom, and many of your patients will know more about their individual disease than you carry in your head. Your job has changed so that you are now your patient's medical interpreter. The Internet has torn up the rules, old-fashioned communication strategies are no longer viable, shared decision making is a must, and in our view concordance rules. Read on.

Reference

Blackburn DF, Swidrovich J, Lemstra M. Non-adherence in type 2 diabetes: practical considerations for interpreting the literature. *Patient Prefer Adherence.* 2013; 7: 183–9.

CHAPTER 3

Different types of patient

- The same words will often mean different things to different people.
- Medical words are confusing and frightening to patients.
- Patients are people, and they are all different.
- What works for one patient probably won't work for another.
- What is most important is what matters to patients.

The health belief model

This is the most researched and validated description of patients' beliefs about health and related matters, and it has five main elements:

1 People's interest in their health and the degree to which they are motivated to change it (health motivation) vary enormously.

2 When considering specific health problems, people think very differently about how likely they are to be affected (perceived vulnerability). For example, people who think that they are at high risk of developing lung cancer are more likely to follow advice about giving up smoking than those who do not think they are at risk.

   If a patient already has a health problem, their perceived vulnerability relates to the degree to which they believe in the diagnosis and its possible consequences. For example, suppose that a patient is diagnosed in the gastroenterology clinic as having irritable bowel syndrome, and it is suggested that tension may be contributing to the condition. If the patient is convinced that pelvic inflammatory disease and not tension is the cause, they are unlikely to adhere to the proposed management plan. This disbelief in what they are told may not be explicit and needs to be searched for. They do not regard themselves as being susceptible to tension, and they therefore conclude that there must be another cause. Their friend was diagnosed with pelvic inflammatory disease and had very similar symptoms, so the doctor must be wrong.

3   Patients vary in how dire they believe the consequences of contracting a particular illness or of leaving it untreated (perceived seriousness) would be.

Heart disease or lung cancer may seem to be a very remote possibility to a 16-year-old girl who is starting to smoke because of peer pressure. Her attitude may be: 'And anyway by the time I get to 40 they will have a cure for it, won't they?'

On the other hand, the publicity about skin cancer resulting from sun exposure has meant that, in recent years, anxious patients have flocked to doctors with a wide range of minor skin blemishes. Peter used to see one such patient in almost every surgery. Most people regard cancer as very serious, and some, if they suspect it, may even be too frightened to go to the doctor. Particularly sad examples of this, which unfortunately are still not uncommon, include older women with slowly growing fungating carcinomas of the breast. Fortunately, young men with testicular growths do appear to have benefited from the publicity about testicular cancer, and they now seem more likely to attend than was previously the case.

4   Patients weigh up the advantages and disadvantages of taking any particular course of action. They do not necessarily take all of the relevant considerations into account, but they make an evaluation of the perceived costs and benefits nonetheless. This cost–benefit analysis is unique to each individual, and can be influenced by outsiders, including doctors. However, in order to influence the equation in the patient's favour, those factors that are already included by the patient need to be known by the doctor. Consider Mrs Arthur and the possibility of ^{131}I treatment. Her fear that radiation would prevent her from conceiving might stop her complying with the treatment because in her own mind the risks of treatment outweigh the benefits. Thus it becomes imperative for the doctor to seek out such fears and talk them through with her.

5   Patients' beliefs do not already exist in a pre-packaged form. They are prompted or created by a number of stimuli and triggers (cues to action), such as a physical sensation, what Granny said, a

television programme or what has just happened to the man down the road.

The health belief model emphasises what we have already discussed. People are generally engaged in a struggle to understand what is happening to them as well as what might happen. Different people try to resolve these dilemmas in different ways. Each person's belief system is of course unique, but it is strongly influenced by race, culture, religion and the immediate society. A poor Chinese farmer will have a very different health understanding to a German banker, but so will people living in the same environment. There will be little similarity between the health understanding of a Geordie miner and that of a black Rastafarian, both living in Newcastle. There are major differences between people in different strata of the same society, and the differences are often still considerable within the same social group.

The health belief model threw up another concept, namely locus of control.

Locus of control

This is jargon for how we explain to ourselves what is likely to happen to our health. Using this idea we can divide the human race into three types of people.

The internal controller

This type of person believes that fundamentally they are in charge of their own future health. In other words, what happens to their health is largely the result of their own actions. This is the organically obsessed, vitamin-swallowing, fitness freak brigade – those diligent humans who digest every morsel of health-related news from the *Guardian* or *Telegraph* health page. They will not have an aluminium pot in the house for fear of Alzheimer's disease, and they are to be found sweating in health-food shops, rummaging for the elixir of life, having just jogged five miles to get there. There are certain implications for this type of believer, not least that they tend to get very cross if they do get ill. To spend 20 years abstaining from the good things in life in order to keep one's cholesterol level below 4 mmol/litre and then still have a coronary at the age of 55 results in a very unhappy and disillusioned human being.

As far as communication is concerned, this type of person likes explanations, dialogue and Socratic inquiry (discussion between individuals based on asking and answering questions to stimulate critical thinking and to illuminate ideas). They want to be involved in decisions about their health and they want to know what is happening. The medical arguments and explanations do not necessarily need to be rational. This group is enthusiastic about alternative medicine and, let's face it, a great many medical explanations are at best dubious and sometimes downright wrong. However, if the explanations are convincing the internal controller will accept them.

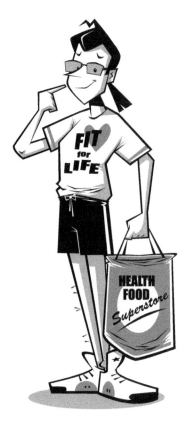

The fussy internal controller

The external controller

This type of person is the opposite of the internal controller. They do not believe that they have any control over their health. What will be will be. They are fatalists. A good example is the 'bullet with my name on it' type of person who can be found down at the local pub expounding their theories as to why these dietary, high-exercise, low-fat and no-alcohol theories much loved by the medical profession are rubbish:

> My grandfather lived to be 95 and he smoked 10 large King Edward cigars a day, washed down with a bottle of Martell. He had clotted cream with everything and was shot in bed with his 25-year-old mistress by her jealous husband.

In Peter's career the most explicit external controller he ever met was a fortyish, unfit mechanic with an expanding paunch who was complaining of feeling rather run down. Among other things, when gently enquiring about exercise and his proclivity towards it the patient knew immediately what Peter was trying to say:

> You're not talking about jogging, are you, doc? I'm not for that at all. Look, I reckon in this life God gives you a certain number of heartbeats and I'm buggered if I'm wasting any of mine running round in bloody circles on wet Sunday mornings!

External controllers are not keen on Socratic dialogue, or at least not as far as their health is concerned. He (or less commonly she) wants to be told what to do and then to ignore the advice or not as the case may be. He is not really much into involvement, and takes little or no interest in the media obsession with health matters. Curiously, research in this field suggests that people with an external locus of control are more likely to be influenced by authoritarian and overly simplistic poster campaigns, much practised by well-intentioned, often government-funded organisations, exhorting people to avoid a variety of pleasurable but possibly dangerous activities.

It is most important for us to remember that the form of communication that will work best with the internal controller will not work well with the external controller. Now we come to the third type of person.

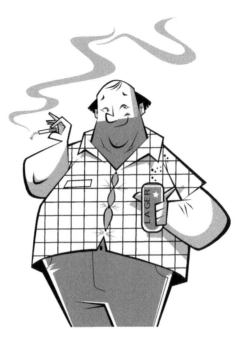

The fat fatalist

The powerful other

This type is quite different from the other two. They do not believe that they are in control of their own health, nor are they fatalists. They believe that *you* are in charge of their health.

> I have this terrible cough, doctor. I know it's not related to my smoking because I have been doing that a long time and it has never bothered me. I'd like you to give me something to stop it.

Doctors, of course, see a disproportionate number of people of this variety. Many of those individuals who have been described as 'heartsink' patients can be found in this category. A great many of these patients will have overt, or more probably covert, mental health issues.

The powerful others of this world pose another difficult challenge for us doctors. Strategies that involve trying to give such patients more responsibility for their own health are firmly resisted. Getting them involved in deciding how to proceed is also difficult, as powerful others are quite firm about their agenda for the doctor, and they are at their happiest with authoritarian doctors who relieve them of any responsibility for their own health. They are not easily educated, and if their agenda for their health does not coincide with that of the doctor, they will not follow the medical advice that they are given.

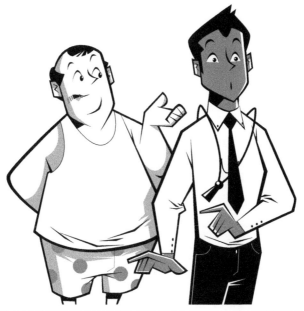

"SO DOC IF I NEED TO STOP THE FAGS AND LOSE SOME WEIGHT WHAT ARE YOU GOING TO DO ABOUT IT?"

Some examples of patients with different loci

Mrs Cheshire is a 50-year-old, 19-stone smoker who hates doctors.

Mrs Cheshire: I've come about my knees, doctor. Something's got to be done. I can't go on like this.

Dr [with an outward sigh and an inner scream]: Mrs Cheshire, you know the problem, you really must lose weight. I can't do anything for those knees till you have at least two stone off. I am sending you to the dietitian and then I want regular weighing by our nurse to keep you on the straight and narrow.

Why doesn't this work? Mrs Cheshire wants relief from pain, a touch of medicinal magic, something fairly easy. She is well aware of her lifelong weight problem, does not think it is that relevant, and certainly does not want the usual doctor response she has heard since her twenties. She thinks that it is her doctor's responsibility to cure her pain, not hers. Unfortunately, you, her doctor, disagree on nearly all counts. Your agendas are mismatched and you think that Mrs Cheshire should take responsibility for her illness and that she can, should and will lose weight, and as a result her knees will improve. You think that the illness is her own fault. This will remain a difficult consultation or series of consultations until one of you is prepared to change agendas. Can you do it? Should you? This woman believes that her health is your responsibility. She is a 'powerful other'.

Here is another common example of a powerful other locus. Miss Moore is a 25-year-old, chronically nervous individual with a set of notes already larger than average, mainly full of minor illness and over-investigated vague complaints. A shortened version of your conversation is as follows.

Miss Moore: Doctor, I am very worried. I am tired all the time and my boyfriend says there must be something seriously wrong with me. Do you think it is my virus again?

Dr [wearily, and with a resigned but worldly-wise air]: No, it's not your virus. We have talked about this before – you worry too much. Stop worrying about yourself and go out and enjoy yourself. There is nothing wrong with you.

You are almost certainly right, but you see her the next evening coming out of your partner's surgery. Why? Perhaps because she wanted you to take on board her fears, take on responsibility for her unwellness, and give her a nice neat little physical illness with a label to wave at her boyfriend. You did not want to do any of this. What else might you have done? You made a good start by recognising her agenda and then overruling it with good reason. Perhaps this was too much of a one-way process. You could recognise her agenda, but she either did not accept or did not wish to be a part of your agenda. There was no negotiation, no 'give and take', no sweetening of the message by dressing it up a bit. A little intelligent sympathy thrown in might help. For example:

> It's rotten feeling tired all the time, everything's an effort. Tell me how it affects you . . . you must find it worrying feeling like this . . . what do you think might be going on? . . . I often find when someone tells me they are feeling like you do that really they are feeling a bit down and miserable. Are you?

How do you cope with another common and difficult consultation? Here we have introspective, fussy Mr Fogarty with a list of minor ailments and a host of strategies for dealing with them, all of which he wants to discuss.

> Do you think I should be taking zinc tablets for my heart? Remember my cholesterol last month was 5.6. Can you remeasure it to see if my walnut and avocado diet is really working?

This man's agenda clearly relates to him being in control of his health – a definite internal controller, but with a desire for a lot of your involvement and a distinct whiff of hypochondria. What is your agenda? Is it to get him out of the room as fast as possible, to help him to educate himself, or to train him to use your services in a reasonable way?

Let us think about your agenda again.

Perhaps you are a well-meaning intervening preventionist, using every opportunity you can to attack obesity, smoking and sloth. Mr Reid, an external controller par excellence, comes to you with a sore throat, smelling of old beer and cigarettes, and knocks over your sphygmomanometer with his swinging gut.

> Come on, doc, out with the penicillin and none of your lectures.

What now? There are myriads of strategies you could try, depending on your inner agenda, but which of them will work? What will satisfy you and yet help your patient?

Influencing locus of control

When Mrs Arthur first went to her family doctor she had prepared her speech, but she did not feel in control of the situation, nor was she fatalistic. She wanted the doctor to take the lead, but she did expect a referral and an explanation. She could not be pigeonholed into any of the three categories described, but perhaps she is closest to a powerful other who, with support, judicious involvement and some education, can be helped to take more control over her worrying illness.

The good thing about locus of control as far as doctors are concerned is that it can be influenced. It is rather like political affiliation – most of us lean to the left or the right, but can sometimes be cajoled to vote the other way. Similarly, locus of control in most people is a tendency, not a fixed aspect of their personality. A further point about external or internal beliefs about health matters is that we humans are not necessarily consistent. For example, I may be at heart more or less a fatalist, but I still buy big chunky cars, believing them to be safer for my family and perhaps for me.

If it is correct that the communication strategy of the medical profession should be directed towards increasing people's tendency to look after their own health and take some responsibility for their health – and we believe that it should – only the internal controllers are going to accept this idea easily. The other 50%–60% of patients are going to need some persuading. However, the effort may be worthwhile for several reasons, not least because it is likely to lead to more patients following more medical advice. In a review of the literature in 2001 it was found that for five behaviours, the odds of healthy behaviour were more than 40% higher among individuals in the internal controller category. Fatalist scores were associated with a reduction of more than 20% in the likelihood of healthy options for six behaviours, while the scores of powerful others showed more variable associations with healthy actions.

Now a cautionary thought about control. Consider type 1 diabetes. Many young female diabetics quickly discover that letting their blood sugar levels rise produces weight loss – high sugar equals small bum. So they make a conscious decision to put their health at risk in the long term in order to obtain a short-term reward. Is this internal control or fatalism? It is certainly common as those of you who deal with diabetes regularly will know already.

If patients all require different styles of communication depending on their locus of control, and research suggests that we doctors have on balance pretty inflexible styles, how are we, as doctors, going to acquire the necessary flexibility without spending all our lives at communication workshops? Heaven forbid.

The answer must be to explore our patients' agendas. If we know their beliefs, and we have an inkling about their locus of control, we can try to follow at least some, if not necessarily all, of their agenda, and talk to them about what matters to them and to us. Communication will therefore become tailored to the individual and will thus automatically become more flexible.

We shall close this chapter with a quote from another doctor who wrote about his own illness in the *British Medical Journal* (Shelford, 2003).

- The information that I want is not that one in ten patients will benefit, but whether I am that one.
- When I return to practice after my treatment, I shall ensure that I focus on the individual in front of me and my traditional consulting skills.

Reference

Shelford G. Risk, statistics, and the individual. *BMJ*. 2003; **327**: 757.

CHAPTER 4

Patient encounter outcomes

When patients meet doctors and some form of communication takes place, they are changed. Not necessarily in ways that doctors may hope for or expect, but some change in understanding does occur. It is important for us to analyse the effects that our contacts with our patients have on their subsequent behaviour and beliefs about health and illness (*see* Figure 4.1).

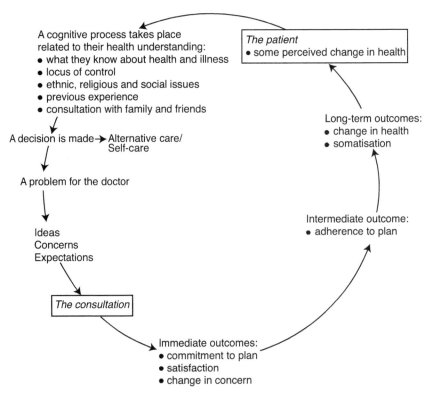

FIGURE 4.1 The patient's learning circle

In the previous chapters we have thought about some of the issues that affect patients' decisions to consult, and what factors make up their health understanding. It is now time to consider the role of doctors as educators in this learning circle. Let us start with the immediate outcomes of a consultation with yourself or another doctor.

Immediate outcomes of the consultation

Commitment to plan

After a patient has consulted you, they come away having made immediate decisions on whether to follow your advice or not. There are many reasons why they may follow your advice. The first and best is that they believe and understand you, and their agenda approximate yours closely. Other reasons include doing what one is told by a respected professional. This may result in the idea that it was not quite what they were expecting, but you are the doctor so they will give it a try. Alternatively, they may just be too frightened to disobey you. There is a halo effect – patients are more likely to take your advice if they like you; they are more likely to like you if you are nice to them. If they like you they are much more likely to see you as trustworthy and wise and so more likely to follow your advice. It's not rocket science, is it?

The problem, as described at the end of Chapter 2, is that 50% or more of patients do not follow our advice closely and are not committed to the plan, most probably because it is our plan and not theirs. Consider the following example.

A 54-year-old man is referred to the cardiology clinic by his GP with a letter saying: 'This man has developed intermittent chest pain over the last 3/12 that has some cardiac features, such as being related to exercise and radiating to his left arm. His resting ECG is normal, BP is 150/85, and I can't find anything obviously wrong. He smokes 20 a day and is a line worker at the car plant. There is no past history of anything significant.'

The clinic is rushed as usual, but you take his history in more detail and examine him thoroughly. Like the GP, you think that there may be an element of angina, and you arrange for him to return for a treadmill test and give him some glyceryl trinitrate tablets to take under his tongue when the pain begins. Later you are surprised to hear that he defaulted from the treadmill test. Why did he default?

In this case, the reason was simple. He thought that you and his GP were investigating the wrong thing. He went to his GP with chest pains, worried that they heralded the onset of oesophageal cancer because his father had presented in the same way. The possibility that the pain might be related to his heart had occurred to him, but it did not correspond to his idea of heart pain. He was confused by the fact that his GP did not mention cancer or ask him about his throat, but he was worried that his GP really did think it was cancer because he sent him to the hospital. He kept his appointment because he thought that the hospital would do tests that would rule out cancer. When he found out that you at the hospital were like his GP – only interested in his heart – he did not feel committed to your plan. He assumed that you were not worried about cancer. He was not concerned about his heart, so he decided to do nothing unless something else developed, in which case he would go back to his GP.

Take asthma as another example. An article published in the journal *Chest* (Horne, 2006) demonstrated that a single question effectively identifies those who don't think their asthma is a chronic disease, and therefore don't manage it as one: 'Do you think you have asthma all the time, or only when you are having symptoms?' In total, 53% of hospital admissions in this study were of the 'no symptoms, no asthma' belief. If you don't really believe that you have the disease, it makes no sense to you to try to prevent it. Among other reasons asthma patients don't take their prophylaxis is fear of long-term side effects worse than their perceived severity of the illness.

Change in concern

The immediate thought most of us have about this is that going to a doctor will reduce concern. However, this is often not true of course. Let us take a simple headache as an example.

In the village in which Peter lives, probably 10 people wake up each morning with a headache, and at the most one or two of them come to the doctor. They usually, but not always, turn out to be the most concerned of the 10 individuals.

The first is a 25-year-old woman who is afraid of her recurrent headaches, and thinks that she probably has a brain tumour. She is hoping to be taken seriously and properly investigated and treated. She has come today because the headache is particularly bad, and she had a row with her boyfriend last night over a television programme about doctors misdiagnosing cancers. It is you who are due to see her and you are rushed. Although you do not discover all of her story you do discover her fear of a brain tumour and see her immense relief at being allowed to talk about it. You examine her thoroughly, including her fundi. This is, of course, intended to be both diagnostic and therapeutic. After discussion, explanation, advice and the offer of a possible follow-up appointment, she leaves you with less concern than when she arrived. Her health understanding has changed a little, but the change is brittle and it will not take much to bring her back.

Your second patient is a 56-year-old banker who says that he is not too concerned about his recent onset of migraines because his mother got them at about this age, but he would like some of those new injections or something like that which he read about in the evening paper. You go through the same routine, but the headache is just too severe when you see him and his obvious distress prompts an urgent (ish) neurological referral. He is grateful but worried.

Imagine that you are now the young F2 doctor in the hospital outpatients. After a brief history you are thinking in migraine mode, but this time you notice a nystagmus to the right and a papilloedema of the left disc with a fuzzy right disc. You are worried and a bit flustered. The banker picks up on your concern, and the urgent need for a brain scan raises his anxiety level considerably.

This is a rare event in medicine – most headaches are not caused by brain tumours. This example is intended to illustrate the rather obvious point that concern can increase after a successful consultation. This point, although not subtle, needs to be borne in mind when reading learned papers about changes in concern.

Let us return to Mrs Arthur. Put yourself in her doctor's seat. When she first came to you, you examined her thyroid thoroughly and did a blood test. You did not mention cancer and neither did she. Did you not mention it because you thought it was cancer and didn't want to frighten her? Was the blood test for cancer? You did say something about going to hospital. Was that in order to see a cancer specialist? Mrs Arthur was not less concerned on leaving.

Remember the interchange at the hospital. How do you think Mrs Arthur's concern changed? If she is very concerned about possible ^{131}I treatment, and nothing you have said has alleviated this concern, her health understanding remains unchanged and she is likely to default.

The effect that the doctor's style can have on the patient's concern is worth repeating. Respected authoritarian physicians have the power to reduce anxiety at the cost of reducing patient autonomy, and this effect is sometimes short-lived. However, giving ill patients too much autonomy can increase their anxiety. This is a difficult equation and it deserves your attention. Sharing information and understanding would seem to be the best compromise, as this approach is most likely to increase autonomy while constraining any increase in concern.

The last point about concern relates to a curve that is well known and much loved by psychologists (*see* Figure 4.2).

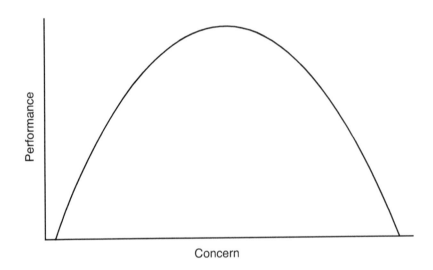

FIGURE 4.2 **Concern measured against performance**

As you can see, performance increases with concern up to a certain point, and then plateaus and falls off. This curve should interest doctors, too. If the anxiety or concern is too great, patients will not do what it is in their best interests to do. This may be why showing rotting cancerous lungs in bottles to smokers is not usually a very effective technique for helping them to give up. It pushes the majority over the top of the curve. Too great a fear of cancer freezes patients into inertia, and usually also stops them hearing what you are saying. On the other hand, a small decrease in concern may put them on peak performance to enable them to face the rigours of the treatment. This is a simple but very important curve.

Here is another important diagram for you to consider, the DiClemente cycle of readiness to change (Figure 4.3). This was developed in the late 1980s to explain smoking cessation behaviour, but it does explain a lot of other behaviours too.

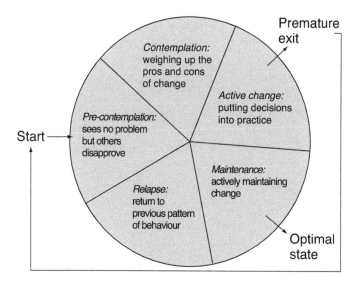

FIGURE 4.3 DiClemente cycle of readiness to change. (Adapted from Prochaska JO, DiClemente CC. Stages and processes of self-change in smoking: toward an integrative model of change. *J Consult Clin Psychol.* 1983; **51**(3): 390–5.

People in the pre-contemplative phase will never quit and those in the contemplative/preparative stage won't either, no matter how concerned they are, unless they can move on to the active change stage.

Satisfaction

This is a commonly measured factor in many articles about doctor–patient communication. The simple equation is high satisfaction = good, and low satisfaction = bad. However, as usual, life is not quite that straightforward. Many health messages are not particularly satis-fying, even if a jury of peers would concur with them. The continuing craze for lifestyle advice, enhanced in the UK by a payment system that reinforces such doctor behaviour, is an obvious example. The patient comes to her GP with a cough and is told to stop smoking, lose weight, have a cervical smear, have her breasts examined and her cholesterol measured, and is then told that she cannot have any cough mixture prescribed. To a large section of the community this may be profoundly unsatisfying, but to the majority of the profession this would now be seen as good practice and certainly lucrative.

There is an easy way to satisfy most patients, and that is to give them what they want. Most alternative therapies work on this prin-ciple. The traditional 'Baked Bean' healing strategy works on the principle that the healer always has an answer and always satisfies the patient:

- My dear, I am glad you are improving. Let's increase the dose of the Baked Beans.
- I'm sure we can help you if we just cut the dose by a tiny amount.
- Don't worry that you have not improved. Let's use the very special sun-dried African Beans that have been hand-picked in the Kalahari.

Thus there is either the right dose, too much, too little or the wrong sort. Medically trained doctors are not immune from this behaviour, but they tend not to be as good at it.

In some cases, especially in those patients in real emotional dis-tress, they themselves don't seem to know what they want, and we doctors keep asking them in the hope we can do something useful without either side knowing what that might be.

The fact that patients often want treatments such as unnecessary antibiotics, excessive time, more of you than you can spare, dubious operations and so on means that the goal of only satisfying patients is a poor one. We need more integrity than that. Again, it becomes obvious that patient satisfaction is a subtle measure and needs to be interpreted carefully.

Some facts about satisfaction are clear. A patient's satisfaction with the consultation is strongly influenced by the amount of informa-tion that they are given. A 1998 review of over 40 studies of patient satisfaction showed that information provision by the doctor was positively associated with patient satisfaction, as was patient information giving, although high levels of closed questions seemed to produce more negative results. Unsurprisingly, doctors' friendliness, courtesy and expression of warm and positive feelings in consultations were positively associated with patient satisfaction, whereas the expression of negative feelings (irritation, anger, etc.) was associated with patient dissatisfaction.

In 1997, in a primary care study of 716 consultations involving a sore throat, Little and colleagues (2001) demonstrated that patients who were more satisfied got better more quickly, and satisfaction was strongly correlated with how well the doctor dealt with the patient's concerns. They went on to point out that this was not easy.

Thus it seems that satisfying our patients is important because the evidence shows that satisfied patients are more likely to follow medical advice. There is little evidence that time makes much difference, but communication and style do. It seems to be the case that warm, friendly doctors are more likely to satisfy patients than cold, business-like ones. In the jargon, 'positive affect' works well. It also appears that doctors talking too much reduces satisfaction, whereas the sense of being listened to and understood increases it. Therefore it is really not difficult – patients like doctors who smile at them, are friendly and actively listen to them, and within this framework they will then accept some of the less pleasant health messages without becoming fed up.

Intermediate outcomes of the consultation: patient concordance, compliance or adherence

There is a difference between the 'commitment to plan', immediate decisions about adherence and the full follow-through to complete the course. Defaulting can occur at any of these stages. The poor uptake of medical advice remains a major challenge to our profession, but it could be argued that within many patients' health understanding there lurks a healthy scepticism about medical advice, and that if we as doctors really do wish to influence our patients to do what we think is good for them, we had better be very certain that we are right.

The patient is more likely to adhere to treatment if they understand and believe the explanation. Some patients will adhere simply because it is a doctor who has told them to. Most will adhere if their own understanding seems to match that of the doctor and their agenda is shared – this is what is meant by concordance. A shared understanding should be a general professional goal. A whole issue of the *British Medical Journal*, entitled 'From compliance to concordance' (2003), was devoted to this topic. The most in-depth analysis of the adherence, concordance or compliance debate is to be found in a report published in 2005 by the National Co-ordinating Centre for NHS Service Delivery and Organisation (NCCSDO), available on their website (www.nets.nihr.ac.uk/__data/assets/pdf_file/0009/64494/FR-08-1412-076.pdf).

There is a fascinating area that we doctors know very little about, namely what lessons our patients learn from whether they follow our advice or not (*see* Table 4.1).

Table 4.1 The effect of adherence on understanding

	Patient gets well	Patient does not get well
Patient adheres to treatment	A	B
Patient does not adhere to treatment	C	D

Around 99% of patients act rationally in terms of their own health beliefs which, however, may not themselves be rational. For example, patient A goes to the doctor wanting penicillin for her sore throat. She is given the antibiotic, gets better and has her health belief confirmed – that penicillin cures sore throats. Patient B does exactly the same thing but does not get better. What lessons has he learned? That penicillin does not cure sore throats? That it was not a 'strong' enough antibiotic and that the doctor was ineffective in choosing the right one ('I've always had the green ones before – these red ones are useless')? That the doctor was right all the time and it was a virus that did not respond to penicillin? That there may be something very serious which the doctor missed? That this doctor is no good and that he will try a different one next time? And so on. There is another possibility with patient B, namely partial compliance. He might be one of the third of patients who take a few pills here and there, but not enough to achieve adequate blood levels (but he may still think that he has followed the doctor's instructions).

What about patient C? He only came for a sick note but was given tablets that he did not want and did not take, and he got better ('I don't know what they teach doctors at medical school, always giving pills for no good reason'). Or what about patient D? She was given penicillin but did not take it because it had given her thrush last time. Now she feels both unwell and guilty. If she goes back to the doctor she might well lie about taking the tablets. These are just some examples of the types of messages that our patients get from whether they do or do not take our advice. How many of these types of messages are we aware of?

Let us go back to Mrs Arthur and put her in each of these boxes; we'll assume that she has a borderline toxic goitre.

In Box A, treatment with ^{131}I is agreed upon. Mrs Arthur's fears about infertility are dispelled, and she complies with the treatment, which is unpleasant but she has been prepared for it. She feels a little better and is grateful for your attention. She still worries about the lumps but is now more likely to accept any further recommendations, such as an operation.

In Box B, she has an unpleasant reaction to the treatment and feels quite poorly. She is totally unprepared, having been given little or no explanation of what the treatment entails, and she is horrified that she had to stay in a small side-ward away from everyone else, and that even her husband was only allowed to see her through a leaded hatch. No one really talked to her during the three unpleasant days she spent in the hospital, and her food was taken away by staff wearing masks and rubber gloves. She is now more convinced than ever that she will definitely be infertile, and she wonders whether you have made an incorrect diagnosis or whether your management was wrong. She is not happy with the hospital and may default any further follow-up.

In Box C, she refuses to come for ^{131}I treatment because of her fears. Anyway, she feels fine now and she thinks that you ordered a dangerous and unnecessary treatment. She has little faith in your opinion that she does or does not need an operation. She may go back to her GP for their opinion, but the GP is also at fault in her view for sending her to that hospital in the first place.

In Box D, Mrs Arthur refuses to come for ^{131}I treatment for the same reasons as in Box C, she but finds herself losing more and more weight. She becomes increasingly frightened but is afraid to call her own GP because she has not followed medical advice.

Of course, the changing pattern of her illness can easily move her from box to box, constantly altering what she is learning from these experiences. Her health understanding will be changed by each meeting with her doctors and by the outcomes of those meetings.

A major problem with communication between doctor and patient concerns the different frames of reference. Doctors are taught scientifically, learn thousands of new words and have models of disease imprinted in their brains. Patients are not like this. Both doctors and patients have reasons for believing and doing what they do – the trouble is that these reasons are different. For example, consider hypertension, a doctor's disease if ever there was one. Until the advent of cheap electronic machines, only professionals could diagnose this condition. Doctors insist to their patients that high blood pressure produces no symptoms and can only be effectively treated by regular medication and frequent monitoring. This is the concept of the asymptomatic risk factor. Most patients cannot understand this approach, and use more obvious folk explanations to help them to cope with what they perceive to be an illness. The result is the adherence nightmare alluded to earlier. Most patients think that hypertension is a description, and take their medication depending on how they feel. If they are feeling headachy, a bit tense and edgy, to them it is obvious that they are hypertensive and need to take their tablets, but on days when they are feeling serene and relaxed it is obviously not necessary to take the tablets. This is all quite logical, but it is using a non-medical frame of reference.

We know more about the way people think since the first edition. For one thing Nobel Prizewinning Daniel Kahneman's *Thinking, Fast and Slow* (2011) has appeared, summarising and expanding on the research of the last 20 years into human psychology. You have to read it. He describes our inbuilt tendency to jump to conclusions and then to look for facts that will confirm these hastily reached opinions. He calls this 'confirmation bias'. Doctors often do this without thinking when we make a diagnosis and we must actively force ourselves to consider other possibilities. Patients do this too – during a conversation with you they may receive a message that you may or may not have meant, but in the subsequent dialogue and after leaving the consultation they will continue to search for evidence that confirms their initial conclusion. This is of course quite the opposite of the testing hypothesis that tries to disprove a theory. It turns out most of us human beings seek data that is compatible with the beliefs we already hold.

Whether or not the patient adheres to the treatment leads to the final outcome in the patient's learning circle. As Webb and Stimson (1975) pointed out:

> The crucial paradox . . . is that in the consultation the doctor makes the treatment decisions; after the consultation, decision-making lies with the patient.

Shared decision making

A great deal of research over the last two decades has confirmed that most, but by no means all, people the world over prefer joint decision making rather than either delegating the decision to the doctor or deciding alone.

In 1990, Lesley Fallowfield studied a cohort of women with breast cancer who were treated by three groups of surgeons – one group whose policy favoured mastectomy, a second group that favoured breast conservation, and a third group that offered a choice of treatment (Fallowfield *et al.*, 1990). There was considerable psychiatric morbidity postoperatively at 3 and 12 months after treatment in all three groups, and there were no differences between the patients who had had a mastectomy and those who had not. However, the patients who were treated by the surgeons whose policy was to offer the patient a choice, including those who for clinical reasons in fact had no choice, showed significantly reduced anxiety and depression compared with the other two groups. More recently, Brian McKinstry, a clever Scottish GP, showed video vignettes of five different presenting conditions to patients (McKinstry, 2000). He found that patients vary in their desire for involvement in decision making, and that this variation depends on the presenting problem, shared decision making being preferred for psychological problems, but the more ill they were or the more physical the problem, the more patients desired a directed approach. Higher social class and educational level were, unsurprisingly, associated with an increased desire for involvement. The variations were very large, making it imperative for doctors to determine for individual patients how much involvement in decision making they want.

Shared decision making is not easy for doctors or patients, but it can and should be achieved in the majority of encounters. Psychological problems can pose a particular difficulty, however. Mild to moderate ones often lend themselves to a sharing approach, but the severely mentally ill may be unable or unwilling to accept any involvement. We will consider some of the difficulties in achieving shared decision making later in the handbook.

Long-term effects of the consultation: change in health

We all try to make sense of changes in our health, and we tend to link them to changes that preceded them. For example, a patient with a bad cold may come to believe that a large tot of Glenmorangie is the best solution if improvement follows in the morning. Another patient may quickly come to believe that antibiotics cure colds if the doctor prescribes them with little explanation. Both of these learned beliefs are in the realms of superstition, and neither is helpful to either the patient or the doctor.

In chronic illness the steady drip of recurrent consultations may build up helpful or unhelpful health strategies; for example, asthma patients addicted to their inhalers, diabetic patients with bizarre dietary beliefs, hypertensive patients who are afraid to take exercise, and so on. Ultimately, we doctors probably play only a small role in influencing our patient's health behaviour, with the Internet, newspapers, family and friends playing a much larger role. All the more reason to try to get the maximum impact from what influence we do have.

Look again at Table 4.1. What other superstitious beliefs can patients develop?

Somatisation

This can be both a presenting complaint and an outcome of the consultation, and is an area that doctors are now beginning to give the attention it merits. The word is ugly and obscure, but it refers to the tendency of patients to create physical symptoms out of emotional responses. Patients don't generally do this consciously; it usually represents an inability or unwillingness to articulate psychological distress. It is quite commonly seen in children. For example, nine-year-old Joshua is taken to the GP after complaining of tummy pain every day before school for two weeks. Examination and blood tests are normal. Mum is subsequently called in to discuss a bullying problem the teacher has recently uncovered centred on her son. Once this issue is resolved the pain goes away.

The degree of individual's insight into this behaviour varies. Some may feel that only physical symptoms will elicit help or sympathy. Others simply have no internal mechanism for processing emotions and are unaware their symptoms are a manifestation of psychological distress. People with learning disability or personality disorder may be especially prone. There is some evidence people who somatise have abnormal pain thresholds and are primed to pay more attention to their physical sensations. They are also more likely to try to link their symptoms together into a single (typically more serious) condition where others would probably dismiss many mild sensations as entirely irrelevant.

This process can be aided and abetted by doctors strenuously trying to make sense of a mass of complaints, and then creating a label which imprints into our patient's mind and then is very difficult to dispel. Patients who somatise their symptoms seem to be less able to talk openly about their emotions, and they often present with woolly, rambling stories linked to fixed, if odd, physical symptoms. They also tend to have an external locus of control. Most people have episodes involving physical complaints that are not explained by organic disease. Low-grade somatisation is common, especially in primary care (1 in 20 patients), and was found to account for at least 20% of the workload of general practitioners in one study conducted in 2003. Effective strategies for managing somatisation are needed that are not too complex for non-psychiatrists. More of this later.

Look again at the patient's learning circle in Figure 4.1. In what areas are your interventions likely to influence your patient's health understanding? Remember that your chance to influence this understanding will not arise very often. With some notable exceptions, patients do not consult with doctors all that frequently. This is particularly true of young and middle-aged men. This is, of course, one more reason why we have relatively little input into the health understanding of most of our patients.

References

Fallowfield LJ, Hall A, Maguire GP, *et al.* Psychological outcomes of different treatment policies in women with early breast cancer outside a clinical trial. *BMJ.* 1990; **301**: 575–80.

From compliance to concordance. *BMJ.* 2003; **327**(7419).

Horne R. Compliance, adherence, and concordance: implications for asthma treatment. *Chest.* 2006; **130**(1 Suppl): S65–72.

Horne R, Weinman J, Barber N, *et al. Concordance, adherence and compliance in medicine taking.* 2005. Available at: www.nets.nihr.ac.uk/__data/assets/ pdf_file/0009/64494/FR-08-1412-076.pdf (accessed 28 March 2014).

Kahneman D. *Thinking, Fast and Slow.* New York: Farrar, Straus and Giroux; 2011.

Little P, Everitt H, Williamson I *et al.* Observational study of effect of patient centredness and positive approach on outcomes of general practice consultations. *BMJ.* 2001; **322**: 908–11.

McKinstry B. Do patients wish to be involved in decision making in the consultation? A cross sectional survey with video vignettes. *BMJ.* 2000; **321**(7265): 867–71.

Prochaska JO, DiClemente CC. Stages and processes of self-change in smoking: toward an integrative model of change. *J Consul Clin Psychol.* 1983; **51**(3): 390–5.

Stimson GV, Webb B. *Going to See the Doctor.* London: Routledge & Keegan Paul; 1975.

CHAPTER 5

How you feel is as important as what you know

The doctor's circle of understanding

This is, of course, the other side of the patient's circle. However, there is a big difference between the two. Most patients do not go round the circle all that often, whereas doctors are going round it all the time. Most doctors see between 2000 and 6000 patients each year. How many do you see? We are often told about learning from experience. Most doctors quite quickly have a lot of experiences with patients, but how much do they learn from these experiences?

Of course you now live in the forced age of the reflective practitioner with your e-portfolios, and if this helps you to learn useful lessons from day-to-day encounters with your patients so much the better. But for some this governmental exhortation to learning can just be downright irritating and not a little demotivating. The trick really is to find the right experiences to reflect upon. The diagram below (Figure 5.1) is useful, having identified the patient/consultation which intrigues you.

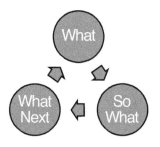

FIGURE 5.1 Reflecting on experiences

The doctor's circle of understanding can be represented as shown in Figure 5.2.

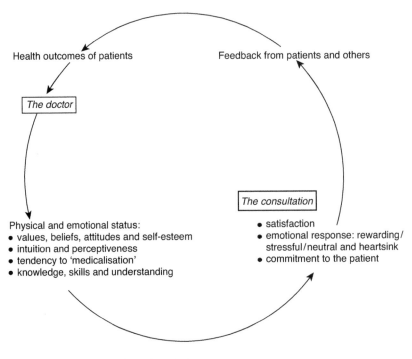

FIGURE 5.2 The doctor's learning circle

Physical and emotional status

How we feel affects how we consult. If you have a feverish cold and still find yourself at work, it can be very difficult to think straight and to make decisions, and when it is apparent that most patients are feeling better than you are, some of your motivation will evaporate. It is obvious that we consult better when we are well, but many doctors, driven by inner goals, soldier on long after the point when it would be better for their patients if they stopped.

Emotional health is more subtle and more insidious. Doctors have a very high incidence of alcoholism, depressive illness and chronic stress disorders. The stiff-upper-lip, lonely, evangelistic medical credo forces them to carry on against the odds, rarely seeking help from colleagues, as this is perceived as a sign of weakness. However, at last the profession is beginning to wake up to the emotional needs of doctors. If you feel yourself becoming emotionally stressed, talk about it with friends, and try to seek help sooner rather than later.

There is also the issue of how patients make us feel, and our response to that feeling. The ability to recognise this process can be helpful. Patients who make us feel the need to rescue them will elicit a different response from us to patients who make us feel like we have failed them, and this can lead to different management. Psychiatrists use the term counter-transference, an old-fashioned and off-putting word. However, the outmoded terminology actually masks a recognised biological process. Humans (and other animals for that matter) are wired to communicate and respond to emotions automatically and usually subconsciously. If we are able to recognise our own emotional responses to an interaction, this can tell us something profoundly useful about the person in front of us who invoked them. This can be especially helpful when dealing with particularly distressed patients who invoke strong responses in us. Understanding this process can help us avoid falling into roles the patient may unconsciously be making us adopt (acting like a parent, being overly punitive, crossing boundaries).

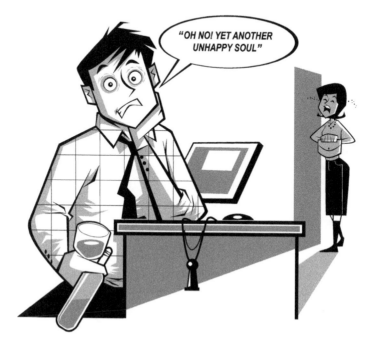

We don't like to admit it but sometimes we are actually afraid of our patients. A study on outpatient consultations in Norway (Mjaaland *et al.*, 2011) found that hospital doctors actively avoided exploring negative emotions expressed by patients, particularly relating to their concerns. There may have been many reasons for this, including fears about lack of time, lack of knowledge or insufficient confidence to deal with emotional responses. Do you find yourself steering conversations with patients away from emotional subjects?

Values, beliefs, attitudes and self-esteem

Like patients, we bring to our consultations a set of beliefs, moral values and attitudes that are derived from our own upbringing, culture and experience. These thinking and feeling patterns will influence how we consult with our patients. A few simple examples will serve to illustrate this point.

- If I am an atheist, I am less likely to suggest to a dying patient that they should seek solace in God.
- If I believe in the total sanctity of human life, I am virtually never going to recommend a termination of pregnancy or be involved in discussions about euthanasia.
- If I am politically left of centre, free market health service policies may be anathema to me, and I may work in such a way as to demonstrate my disapproval.
- If I believe that unsolicited lifestyle advice is an intrusion into personal liberty, I am not going to offer it very often, or if I do it will be half-hearted and only given because I get paid for it.
- If I believe that my job is to diagnose serious illness, I am likely to believe that my patients' ideas and worries are relatively trivial.
- If I believe that it is better for patients with serious illnesses to be protected from the whole truth, I will withhold information.
- If I believe that the patient's ideas and concerns are important, I will seek them out.

And so on.

Think about your own beliefs and attitudes. How do they affect the way in which you consult or feel about patients? Can you compromise from time to time? Can you justify your attitudes to yourself? Can you justify them to your peers? Would you say that you have an accepting attitude with regard to your patient's point of view and beliefs, or is it more a judgemental attitude which equates your patient's worth with their knowledge and beliefs, and places your point of view above theirs?

Our self-esteem is relevant. What is our status? How important is status to us and how motivating is it? Do we need to be powerful in order to protect our fragile self-esteem? Do you consult with patients in such a way as to enhance your own self-esteem, or is this not too important a factor to you? How important is the approval of your friends and peers? How do you maintain your self-respect when dealing with your patients? How do you develop self-confidence? Think about it.

Intuition and perceptiveness

These are both God-given and learned. Intuitive medical behaviour may be based on experience – effectively a synaptic short-circuit – but some doctors are better at it than others. Usually, the more intuitive doctors are the more experienced ones. When you are learning, do not trust too much to intuition. Go back, recheck and try to trace the intuitive pathway until you can follow the logical thread.

Expert intuition is often no better than a simple algorithm, although it can be better than this if steered in a structured direction to consider all the relevant information. We must avoid 'what you see is all there is' or, in other words, making hasty decisions based only on the obvious information in front of us without searching for all the other relevant factors. (For more detail see *Thinking, Fast and Slow* [Kahneman, 2011].)

Without feedback on the outcomes following our decisions we cannot really know how well we are doing. Intuitive expertise is more likely to develop when we get immediate and repeated feedback. We can all accrue intuition in the form of rules we learn from repeated experience. So anaesthetists develop intuition more readily than psychiatrists! However, the cognitive illusion of validity means that even if we were faced with the fact that our decision making was hardly better than blind guesswork, we would undoubtedly continue to believe that there was merit in our judgements. Our decisions are probably more related to stereotyping and the halo effect than we realise.

System 1 and 2 and effortful thinking

We have a limited capacity for effortful thinking (most of us cannot solve a complex puzzle while negotiating a busy roundabout).
*Thinking about a patient's unconscious communications requires
effort!*

System 1 and system 2 are metaphors for different cognitive
processing abilities. System 1 is our automatic brain, which offers up
information it feels is relevant and associated with the issue at hand
without any effort on our part. Short cuts like this are inbuilt into
humans. We are designed to make associations, to create a coherent
picture, to make sense of things. Our system 1 offers us this even
when the evidence it is based on is incomplete or inaccurate. We don't
choose to experience an emotional reaction or a perception; they
just happen. System 2, on the other hand, is conscious, effortful and
has the role of endorsing or discarding the information presented to
it by system 1. We perform better at tasks requiring system 2 input
when we have adequate glucose, are not distracted, take time, and
are frowning (yes, really!). Perceptiveness is a system 2 process; it is
effortful and must be learned.

Sherlock Holmes remains one of the finest role models, based by
Conan Doyle on a senior medical figure in Edinburgh. Consulting
with and examining patients forms the basis for developing your
perceptive skills. Really seeing them, truly hearing what they say (or
do not say) and understanding them and their context are the flesh
on those bones.

Tendency to 'medicalisation'

Ivan Illich, the Austrian philosopher, visionary and perceptive critic
of Western healthcare, coined this deliberately ugly term to describe
the medical tendency to organise vague symptoms into categories, and
to label these categories and so produce a disease that can then be
approached in the traditional medical manner. This tendency is particularly obvious in the medical handling of the everyday emotional
trauma that all human beings experience. For example, unhappiness
is a human condition, whereas 'depression' is a disease that can be
treated with antidepressants.

Labelling people creates illness. People who are found to have mild
hypertension and who are told this fact suddenly have more sickness

absence, have a higher incidence of impotence, cut down their participation in sport by over 50%, have double the incidence of panic attacks, and view themselves differently. This is *before* any possible drug side effects are manifested. Think about this for a moment. This means that all diagnoses have costs. To suddenly turn a normal patient into a 'hypertensive' is not a neutral event. Such a patient's perception of himself or herself has been altered quite markedly for the worse. Therefore you must be quite certain that your diagnosis and subsequent intervention are going to outweigh the harm done.

There is also the medicalisation of daily living – encouraging people to consult doctors about the minor vagaries of life and health, a creeping stripping of personal autonomy, and the gradual creation of a society that is dependent on the medical professions for all wisdom on diet, exercise, lovemaking and everyday existence. In April 2002, a whole edition of the *British Medical Journal*, entitled 'Too much medicine', was devoted to the dangers of creeping 'medicalisation'. Three quotes from this edition are given below:

> If you stop smoking, drinking and having sex you don't actually live longer, it just feels longer.
>
> Clement Freud

> If we choose to 'medicalise' the whole of our existence, we realise that life is a pathological process, a sexually transmitted terminal illness whose prognosis can be predicted at the moment of birth.
>
> Michael O'Donnell

> I don't smoke or drink. I don't stay out late and I don't sleep with girls. My diet is healthy and I take regular exercise. All this is going to change when I get out of prison.
>
> Graffito

If we as doctors subscribe either consciously or unconsciously to this widespread tendency, it will affect both the way in which we consult and the outcomes of those consultations. *A medicalising doctor and a somatising patient are a bad combination.*

Constraints

It is not easy to consult well, and our modern environment can and does make it more difficult. Contracts that reward behaviour geared towards population health improvement strategies discourage the open, patient-centred approach. Time constraints multiply. The fear of a complaint lurks in every meeting. Continuity in primary and secondary care is breaking down. An everyday hospital scenario might be:

> Mrs P wants to talk about her husband's impending gastric resection. It is already 12.30 and you still have 35 of your 60 patients to see, spread all over the hospital. You have already decided to miss lunch. You are the only member of your team here today and you have calculated how long you have to spend with each person. You are sympathetic but know if you stop for half an hour there will be patients who don't get seen at all today and you feel that your primary responsibility has to be to your patients.

However, you only need to watch a few episodes of *24 Hours in A&E* to see that great communication is possible even within extremely short patient interactions, in corridors, with lots of noise and surrounded by chaos, if the doctor cares enough.

True advocacy requires access to resources, but these are often scarce. The weight of patient expectations can be hard to cope with, and the constant uncertainty of diagnosis and prognosis weighs on us all. But don't get too disheartened – there have always been constraints, and if you care you can rise above most of them most of the time.

Knowledge, skills and understanding

This is the area that is traditionally the focus of medical school. It is for our knowledge, and the skills in applying that knowledge, that the public come to us. We learn about diseases and about techniques to diagnose and treat these diseases, and we listen to aphorisms such as 'There is nothing more important than diagnosis, diagnosis and diagnosis.' We slave over sweet-smelling corpses as we search for aberrant nerves, and we learn by rote the mysteries of the Krebs cycle. We are multiple-choiced to the point of exhaustion, and we are taught to learn by an adversarial style of one-upmanship. We feel guilty about reading a novel because we should be reading medicine. There is so much that it is unencompassable, and if we are not careful, in all this knowledge we shall lose our understanding of people and what makes them tick.

We must use our consultations with our patients to increase our knowledge, to hone our skills and most of all to improve our understanding of illness, of people and of ourselves. Then, with all of these strands of ourselves mixed together as our 'givens', we come to the consultation. There is an interaction, a conversation, some laying on of hands – whatever – but at the end of the consultation some things have changed for us as they have for our patients. Let us look at these possible outcomes.

Satisfaction

We all want to do a good job and to take pride in so doing. This affects how we perform. For instance, there is some evidence that doctors who have low job satisfaction prescribe more tranquillisers and antibiotics, and they have shorter consultations. In order to derive regular satisfaction from patient encounters, we need to like what we are doing, have reasonably clearly defined aims, and obtain frequent, supportive feedback that tells us how we are doing and how we can improve. I suspect that not many of us receive much of that type of feedback.

Satisfaction also relates to several internalised goals and the measurement of our achievements against those goals.

> That was a good consultation because she came in very unhappy, but I spotted that, I let her cry, and then she told me what was really worrying her.

The goal here is to increase one's perceptiveness in order to increase one's therapeutic potential.

> That was a good consultation because I diagnosed myxoedema.

The goal here is to be a good diagnostician.

> I was satisfied with that consultation because I felt we really did achieve a genuine shared understanding.

This is arguably even harder to achieve in hospital these days when trainees rarely see a patient through their journey and often receive little or no feedback on outcomes, or any gratitude from anyone. It is inevitable that juniors seek satisfaction in other ways, such as through forming alliances with colleagues or just clocking off on time. It is difficult to feel satisfaction from doctoring when you never know whether what you are doing is any use and you rarely see patients get better as a result of something you have done. Think about what some of your own goals are with regard to patients. From what do you derive satisfaction?

Emotional responses

Dealing with people who are seeking your counsel can be immensely rewarding if you find that your knowledge and skills enable you to help them. This can give you a buzz – an emotional high – that is unmatched by most other occupations. However, there is a downside, too. You will meet many patients whom you cannot help very much, some in great distress. You will meet some patients and know from the start that the outcome can only be a lingering, painful death. This will be hard for you, and you need to develop strategies to enable you to cope with this emotional pain. Many doctors do this by retreating behind cold, professional veneers, sharing little with their patients, telling them less and effectively 'switching off'. However, there are more effective and less drastic strategies than this.

Helping people to die can be very gratifying if it is done well, especially with patients whom you have grown to know as people. There is emotional pain, but this is tempered by the satisfaction of helping a fellow human being through those last days, weeks or months – sharing knowledge, showing compassion, alleviating pain, facilitating communication with partner and family, using other medical skills to maintain tolerable bodily functions to the end, and not deserting them. Unless they specialise in terminal care, most doctors do not see dying patients very often, so there is no need to develop armour-plated communication techniques. In the vernacular, 'stay loose'.

There are myriads of possible emotional responses to a consultation. Sad patients may make us feel sad. Michael Balint, a Hungarian psychoanalyst who worked for many years at the Tavistock Clinic and founded the genuinely reflective 'Balint Group', suggested that the way patients make us feel is a pretty good guide to how they are feeling (see Balint, 1957). So if you feel angry at the end of a consultation, perhaps your patient was angry as well? Consulting under time pressure, as most of us do, creates its own stresses and frustrations. In a busy clinic, when you are already running an hour late, nice Mrs Jones trying to tell you her life story can wind up your inner spring until your teeth clamp together.

There are also those especially difficult patients, usually frequent attenders with incurable problems, demanding that you do something for them. As mentioned before, this group has been labelled 'heartsink' patients, and most clinics have at least one person in this category. Somehow you will have to learn how to retain a sense of humour and compassion, and to keep too much cynicism at bay. It is true that looking at the list of patients to be seen can, on occasions, produce a sense of pre-consultation gloom. This is one advantage of reaching consultant status – you can pass on such people to your juniors.

There are some patients who would try the patience of a saint, and we all have to find ways of coping with them. There are various strategies for managing really difficult patients. The most important being the First Rule – remember it is the patient who has the problem, not you. Others include goal setting, motivational interviewing, and solution-focused approaches. Pain clinics specialise in such needy and challenging people day in and day out so there must be satisfaction to be gained here somewhere!

You will hear much discussion of 'burnout' and the epidemic of stress affecting doctors. This is a complex issue, but from a communication point of view, as a doctor becomes increasingly fed up and stressed they see more and more of their work as trivial and unrewarding, and a vicious circle develops. Interest in patients as people wanes, their stories are not listened to, their fears remain unexplored, and surgeries become wastelands of sore throats and headaches.

Roger Neighbour, in his illuminating book *The Inner Consultation* (2005), discusses ways in which we doctors can care for ourselves. He calls it 'housekeeping', the point being that unless we can keep ourselves in good trim emotionally, we cease to be effective with our patients, and our personal life will also suffer. You should read his book.

Commitment to the patient

After a consultation, some sort of bond will have been formed. It may be tenuous and fragile or it may be a true contract, with responsibilities on both sides. There has to be some commitment on our part or we fail as carers. Our patients certainly expect us to follow through and to be involved with them. This is the beginning of trust. In our learning circle we shall experience many different levels of commitment. A few examples are listed here.

- The terminally ill young wife with advanced breast cancer at the far end of your ward. You have become very involved with her and her bewildered husband, so much so that you have given them your own phone number so that they can call you at any time when they need you. Now that is commitment.
- The pleasant but chronically anxious schoolteacher with increasing panic attacks. He rings you when you are very busy and asks to see you as soon as possible. You offer him some time when you should be off duty. That shows more commitment.
- There is Mrs Arthur holed up having her iodine treatment. She sends a message asking you to come and talk to her. Do you go? She asks you to contact her husband and explain to him what is happening. Will you do so?

We cannot commit ourselves deeply to every patient with whom we come into contact, or we would be swamped. However, we must give each of them a degree of commitment. It is part of our learning circle to judge the appropriate level of commitment that we need to make to an individual who seeks our help.

Feedback

The feedback that we receive from our patients is haphazard and highly selective. The happy ones come back, write us letters, send us occasional presents, tell us how good we are and make us feel good about ourselves. The patients with whom we have been less successful may never come back. They probably will not contact us at all. Rarely, we might be chastened to hear one of them discussing us in unflattering terms on top of a bus, but usually we just don't hear. This means that feedback from patients is very much distorted in our favour. It is easy to spend one's life in a fool's paradise.

Doctors need unbiased, constructive feedback. The current outbreak of patient satisfaction questionnaires is going some way towards improving this situation, but most of the feedback is general, whereas it is the specific feedback that we find most useful.

You live in the age of *Doctor Foster*, *iWantGreatCare*, and other rating websites for doctors. Do you embrace this or does it terrify you? We know many don't register at all or only tend to get the extreme, negative reviews. Interestingly, all the studies show that most patients are more interested in how nice we were to them, and how much we listened than what we actually did. They may throw the pills away, but they will remember the first doctor who seemed to really understand them. They may not get better at all, and we may see this as a negative outcome, but perhaps they won't. Feedback is therefore highly subjective and also dangerous. To be good doctors we do actually need to try to help people in a way that is meaningful for them. If they didn't really want the tablets why did we prescribe them?

Similarly, you may do exactly what a patient asks of you and still find them dissatisfied with the *way* you did it.

Health outcomes of patients

If our patient gets better as a result of our ministrations, this feeds back into our knowledge store, as does the patient who does not get better. On a mechanistic level we can learn from our various tinkerings what helps and what does not help. We often pretend to be academic, and we live in the increasingly oppressive world of evidence-based medicine, but most doctors will trust their own experience of 10 people on a particular drug more than a clinical trial of 1000 patients. 'I have seen it before and I know that that happens' is a traditional part of the art of medicine. This is not to deride the scientific basis of some of our knowledge, or to belittle the power of the double-blind randomised controlled trial. It is just to acknowledge human behaviour and the power of personal experience. There is the concept of 'cognitive ease', in that we are more likely to make a decision based on something we can easily recall, such as a recent patient's successful outcome, than seek through our memory banks for another solution, such as the data from the latest trial.

Then there are base rates which matter more than we think. Some academics deride our humanistic 'evidence', which typically focuses on outcomes in small numbers of patients, as they point out that such small samples cannot possibly be statistically significant, however much we might want to see a pattern emerging. *But* the story that makes more sense to us will seem overwhelmingly more appealing. How plausible and how likely something is are completely different but easily confused concepts. Our system 2s are lazy and often fail to apply the correct rule unless we force ourselves to examine our thinking critically (and effortfully). Ask yourself: 'How is this one different?' Question the validity of your evidence. When the evidence is weak, stick closer to the base rates.

Table 5.1 What doctors learn from patients' responses to protocols

	Patient gets well	Patient does not get well
Doctor complies with professional protocols	A	B
Doctor ignores professional protocols	C	D

We live in a world of ever more numerous protocols and treatment plans. Remember Table 4.1? We considered the possible conclusions patients might take away from the various situations. Now take a moment to consider what doctors learn from such day-to-day encounters with patients – look at Table 5.1.

For example, the doctor could conclude from experience with patients A and D that recommended protocols are effective, whereas their experience with patients B and C could shake their faith.

Given the variety of influences that determine whether or not patients get well, this feedback is extremely unreliable. It is essentially superstitious – the associations inferred between the doctor's behaviour and its consequences for the patient are not necessarily causal.

Every patient is unique, and this is why medicine is so difficult to teach and to learn. What works for one patient will not work for another. If we observe the outcomes carefully and develop our perception, this will feed back into both our knowledge and our understanding store and will increase our intuitiveness. What we have to take into account in this equation is not just the treatment we gave or the advice that we proffered. We also need to remember the style in which the consultation was conducted, whether it was doctor-centred or patient-centred, relaxed or rushed, and how the relationship was, as all of these factors will affect what happens to our patients.

Look again at the full learning circle in Figure 5.2, and think of five patients you have seen recently. Write down what the outcomes of those consultations were for you, and then think how those outcomes feed back into your 'givens' – the items listed to the left of the consultation.

OK? Done that? Then now it is time to look into the black box to see what the consultation should contain.

References

Balint M. *The Doctor, His Patient and the Illness*. London: Tavistock Publications; 1957.

Kahneman D. *Thinking, Fast and Slow*. New York: Farrar, Straus and Giroux; 2011.

Mjaaland TA, Finset A, Jensen BF, *et al*. Physicians' responses to patients' expressions of negative emotions in hospital consultations: a video-based observational study. *Patient Educ Couns*. 2011; **84**(3): 332–7.

Neighbour R. *The Inner Consultation*. 2nd ed. Oxford: Radcliffe Publishing; 2005.

Too much medicine. *BMJ*. 2002; **342**(7342).

CHAPTER 6

What you need to achieve in a patient encounter or consultation

> You must know more about your patient as a person at the end of the consultation than you did at the beginning.

What follows is not the same as the traditional method of history taking. In some ways it amounts to the same thing, but it is a better method. The focus of this chapter is on the initial clerking, encounter or consultation, but there is advice that will help you with shorter and ongoing interactions with patients. The concepts are rooted in the discussions in the previous chapters, and the model works for all patient encounters in whatever setting. There are four main headings.

1 Discover the reasons for the patient's attendance:
   a understand the patient
   b understand the problem.
2 Share understanding.
3 Share decisions and responsibility.
4 Make effective use of the encounter.

To use an American expression, let us 'unpack' each task in turn.

Discover the patient's issues

Understand the patient

Before you started reading this book it may have seemed obvious in most outpatient clinics why most patients were there. Now we hope it is apparent to you that patients do not come to see doctors because they have liver disease. They come because they perceive that their health has changed, and they have a whole set of beliefs and expectations relating to this change in health. On the whole it is doctors who tell them that they have liver disease. So where should we start?

The best bet is usually with the patient.

Listen to the patient describing the reasons for attending

Remember William Osler's dictum to listen to the patient because they are trying to tell you the diagnosis. The simplest way to do this is to let the patient talk, actively encourage their contribution to the consultation, and watch your patient all the time they are talking. Look for cues (both verbal and non-verbal) and try not to interrupt too much. Use your perceptive faculties to hear what they are saying, and try to pick up the message behind the message. We shall discuss some of the effective skills later in the book, but for now just think for yourself how best you would encourage the patient.

There are good reasons for letting the patient have a minute or two of relatively uninterrupted dialogue at the beginning of a consultation. The first is that it often *saves time*. This may be counterintuitive, but it is true. The reasons why letting the patient talk can save time are related first to the patient's agenda and also to yours.

The patient, *and only the patient*, knows the reasons they have come to see you. If you start on your agenda too soon you may never discover the fear of cancer or the fear of the effects of the expected therapy, but more importantly you may not discover what it is that the patient actually wants to know. You may waste 20 minutes testing and reassuring them about a normal cardiovascular system when their actual concern was about oesophageal cancer. The woman with the breast lump who returns after a positive biopsy *needs* to tell you her ideas, her fears and her expectations to help you both plan the best management.

The point about you starting on your agenda too soon is significant. It is well documented that doctors make hypotheses very early on in a consultation – usually in the first 30 seconds, sometimes even earlier. Once you have made a hypothesis (e.g. 'This woman has toxic multinodular goitre'), all of your energies are channelled towards proving that hypothesis (that pesky 'confirmation bias' again). There follows a rapid-fire series of clinical, closed questions directed towards that end, to the exclusion of a broader picture. Another hypothesis will only arise if your clinical search is sterile, or you actively engage your effortful system 2 to search for alternatives. We doctors are very bad at falling into this trap. Many doctors do not even generate differential diagnoses in their head, but just leap to the first diagnosis which suggests itself and ask questions which confirm that. You will gain so much more valuable information by consciously delaying making your first hypothesis for, say, just one minute. Try it. It is hard to do at first but very rewarding.

Establishing your patient's agenda early on also allows you to negotiate the use of time – to agree on what will be dealt with now and what can be left for another day. This is a very important skill to learn early in your career, as it can save so much time and prevent so much unnecessary stress.

Always keep watching your patient, so that you do not miss any cues – verbal or visual. You do not always have to act on them, but ignoring the patient's cues will mean that you will be less effective. A cue is a signal from a patient to a doctor to respond. Cues and responses can be both verbal and non-verbal. Verbal cues may be simply what is said, or they may be what is *not* said and may be related to the tone of voice, facial expression, posture or actions of the patient.

Here are a few examples.

The patient with headaches may say, 'My husband thought I ought to come and see you about these headaches I have been having recently', inviting a response to discuss her husband's concerns.

Or to go back to your consultation with Mrs Arthur in outpatients, you ask, 'Is there anything else worrying you?', to which she replies, 'Er . . . no, I don't think so', while dropping her gaze and nervously fiddling with her handbag. Do you take this denial at face value? You could pick up on her verbal and visual cues and perhaps say, 'There is something, isn't there? Try to tell me what is worrying you.'

Later, while examining her, you ask about previous pregnancies and she says that she has no children, but you notice that her eyes moisten and there is a slight catch in her voice. Do you ignore these cues? Or do you say something like 'You seem a little upset – why is that?' or 'Is becoming pregnant something very important to you?'

As an example of a verbal cue that is not responded to, the patient may say, 'It's my back again', and you only address the present episode, without exploring the previous ones implicit in the cue.

Reflection can be a response to a cue. For example, the patient might say 'and I've felt low this week', and the doctor might reply, 'Low?' Equally, the same cue could be responded to by a later statement by the doctor: 'You mentioned earlier that you felt low. Could you expand on that?'

Other examples include the following:

- 'You seemed upset by . . . Were you?'
- 'I noticed in your records you had . . . last year. Is that still a problem?'
- 'You mentioned your family. What do they think about this?'
- 'Now that was a sigh – what does it mean?'

Picking up on the cues that our patients give us is a skill that all doctors need to develop. These are the signposts to the hidden or not so hidden agendas. No aspiring doctor can hope to be effective or to derive job satisfaction without developing an ability to use cues and having a sense of when to act and when to wait. This takes time to develop, and its absence is one of the commonest weaknesses observed when watching doctors in training talking to patients. In a study published in the *British Medical Journal* (Barry *et al.*, 2000), only 4 of 35 patients voiced all of their agendas in the consultation. The most common unvoiced agenda items were worries about the possible diagnosis and what the future held, ideas about what was wrong, side effects, not wanting a prescription, and information relating to their social context.

Intriguingly, many doctors who seem perfectly able to pick up on such cues in real life seem to switch off this ability when confronted with a simulated scenario like those in postgraduate exams. Perhaps this is an excessive focus on the 'task' to the utter exclusion of all else, or maybe it reflects a lack of confidence. Either way, failing to pick up on patient cues is often (quite rightly) a significant factor in failing exams.

Obtain and use relevant social and occupational information

Why not do this at the beginning, too? At least you can then place your patient in a social context and begin to know a little of them as a sentient human being with a home to go to and, if they are lucky, a job to do. You will need to elicit sufficient details to place the complaint(s) in a social and psychological context, and perhaps to gain some knowledge of the cause(s) of the problem.

You will also need to establish the effect of the illness on the patient's work or home life. We doctors often forget about such effects, but to our patients these may be the main reason for them coming to see us. This is often particularly noticeable in primary care, although it is equally problematic in hospitals. People in beds often seem to merge together after a while and the pressures of busy ward rounds can mean that interactions are brief and perfunctory at best. We advise anyone with a relative in hospital to bring in a photo of them to put by the bed as this definitely helps those of us who work in hospital to remember that this is a real person with a life outside of G7.

Meanwhile, a chain-smoking miner with advanced emphysema may be hoping for some more breath to allow him to walk to the club and to be able to climb the stairs to visit his disabled daughter. The fact that we may not be able to offer more breath, but we know his reasons for coming to us, may help us and him to make a realistic assessment. We can then offer the help of other agencies in providing wheelchairs, stair lifts, home oxygen, and other assistance, while not pretending that we can perform any magic.

There are two ways to look at this task. As continuity of care is decreasing, it is becoming even more important to find out this kind of information in every consultation. In those circumstances where you hope for some continuity of care, each time you obtain some personal information you can regard this as a 'brick' and over time you will build a wall.

Looking at recordings of doctor–patient encounters, it is surprising how often doctors do not seem to be very interested in their patient as an individual. Patients come with sore throats, an attack of thrush, or for a repeat prescription for the pill, and all that happens is a quick transaction. The doctor knows no more about the patient at the end of the consultation than at the beginning. If this is our regular pattern, who are GPs kidding when they call themselves family doctors? Make it a rule to know more about your patient when they leave than you did when they came in. In the 10 years of watching MRCGP videos we saw relatively few 'bricks', which was and remains dispiriting. The MRCGP video exam is no more but the new CSA, and all the other comparable clinical OSCE-style exams are possibly even less encouraging as the stations are so short there is an implicit discouragement of straying too far beyond the task in hand. While pretended empathy and tricks of active listening are rewarded, actually understanding patients and knowing more about them may not be.

Just obtaining the information is not enough – using it is the crux. For example:

- 'So how is the back pain affecting what you do?'
- 'You said that your husband was upset after your mastectomy. Tell me more about how this has affected you both.'
- 'You said things at work are pretty hectic. Do you think that has a bearing on how you feel?'
- 'How do you manage at home?'
- 'This has been a bit of a strain for you, hasn't it? So tell me about it.'
- 'Tell me more about some of the stresses.'

Explore the patient's health understanding

If you have allowed the patient to talk for a while, some of their understanding will have been revealed, but some will need to be actively searched for – their ideas, their fears and concerns, and their expectations. Remember what you read in Chapter 3. You might get an inkling about their locus of control. You must take the patient's health understanding into account in enough detail to ensure that there is a reasonable probability that the consultation will be successful. Remember that the patient is the expert on their own life.

For example, in the case of a patient with headaches, the doctor may say, 'You have had these headaches for a few weeks now, and I was wondering whether you had any ideas yourself as to what they might be due to?' This invites the patient to discuss their health understanding with the doctor, indicating that the doctor is interested and concerned about the patient's understanding of their symptoms.

In its most overt form, it simply requires the doctor to say, after hearing the patient's story, 'What do *you* think it could be?', or something similar. There are few situations where such a question, properly and sensitively asked, is not appropriate. (The obvious exception would be when the patient has already told you; for example, 'I cut my finger this morning while opening a can of beans'!)

If the patient asked, 'Do you think it's an allergy, doctor?' and the doctor replied, 'Certainly not!', or words to that effect, they would not be exploring the patient's health understanding. If, on the other hand, they had replied, 'What do *you* think?' they would be exploring that understanding. Clearly, this task has a large 'attitude' component – that patients' ideas are intrinsically valid and valuable in understanding the nature of their problem.

In the early days it is easy to be put off by replies such as 'I haven't really thought about it; you are the doctor', and so on. These are untruths, as everybody has some health understanding, but direct questioning may not reveal it initially.

Examples of helpful questions include the following:

- 'People usually have some ideas about their illness. What have you been thinking?'
- 'What would be your worst fear?'
- 'What had you been hoping to get out of our meeting today?'

To return to Mrs Arthur again in outpatients, you might ask, 'Is there anything worrying you?' Your train of thought is to rule out an anxiety state as a cause of her symptoms. Mrs Arthur wonders if she should tell you about her fear of cancer, but she decides that would make her look foolish, so she replies, 'No.' This is untrue but well meant. If you accept this reply at face value, your 'history' will be the poorer for it.

Enquire about other problems

The presenting complaint may not be the most important factor to the patient or to you. The patient may be presenting with an acute complaint while also suffering a chronic condition; for example, an acute pneumonia in a diabetic, intermittent claudication in a patient on beta-blockers for hypertension, thyrotoxicosis in a woman with multiple sclerosis, and so on. You must obtain enough information to assess whether a continuing complaint represents an issue that must be addressed in this consultation.

Now to the 'proper' doctor bit.

Understand the problem

Try to define the problem

Having discovered in the patient's words why they have come to see you, you can now form a working hypothesis and start to put some of your clinical pigeonholing skills into operation.

Obtain additional information about critical symptoms or details of the medical history

First, you must obtain sufficient information to be sure that you are unlikely to miss any life-threatening conditions. Second, your verbal investigation should be consistent with your hypotheses, which you have now formed on the basis of information you have just obtained in the consultation. This part is well taught in medical school, but do observe how your chiefs consult. What history-taking short cuts do they use? You may have to learn how to 'take' a full history, but there will be few times in your career when you do not modify what you have learned to be more appropriate to the circumstances.

You must learn to recognise, from what has been said, any potentially 'serious' diagnoses. These would typically include suicidal thoughts in a patient with depression, malignancy in a patient with chronic cough, change in bowel habit, dysphagia or weight loss, and so on. You may achieve this by asking focused, closed questions, such as 'Have you noticed any blood in the stool (sputum, urine)?' or 'Have you ever felt things were so bad you wished you didn't wake up in the morning?'

'Serious' need not mean life-threatening. A child with a cough or otitis media should probably be asked about asthma symptoms, or about their hearing. A person with backache should, unless it was manifestly trivial, be asked about 'red flag' symptoms.

Assess the condition of the patient by physical inspection if appropriate

The examination you choose should be one that is likely to confirm or refute your hypothesis or any other hypothesis that could reasonably have been formed on the basis of the evidence you have so far. This can be a little difficult, as the more experienced and expert you become, the more hypotheses you will be able to generate. A thorough and intelligent examination is required. This next sentence may sound like heresy but – whisper it quietly – some patients only need examining in order to reassure them, to address a specific concern. For example, consider the case of an anxious young woman with intermittent chest pains. The power of the examination and negative ECG is therapeutic, not diagnostic, 99 times out of 100. Most good physicians are aware that if they do not know the diagnosis after talking to the patient, the examination will rarely illuminate it.

Make a working diagnosis

In primary care, detailed clinical diagnoses are uncommon in the sense of the widely used disease model of medicine. The diagnosis becomes a flexible concept to allow the formulation of a rational and appropriate management plan. For example, 'Sore red throat for 3 days? Strep? Virus, patient not ill and not too fussed about antibiotics, just needs reassurance' or 'Recurrent headache with all the characteristics of tension in a chronically anxious frequent attender who will need some strategy or therapy to improve these headaches'.

In hospital, the disease-based formulation is more dominant, but it is dangerously exclusive, as has already been demonstrated. For example, 'Multinodular goitre with hot spots needs more investigation and probably surgery.'

Doctors need to form clinically appropriate working diagnoses on which they can formulate further plans for refinement of the diagnosis if necessary, or on which to base a management plan for their patient.

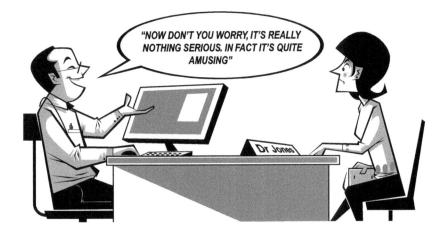

Assess the severity of the presenting problem

You have to use some judgement here. The simplest example is triage – practised by battlefield surgeons and by emergency doctors on Saturday nights. You will have to categorise your patients' problems into types with differing degrees of severity and then treat the individual problem appropriately. On a battlefield you would not treat a man with toothache; in the ED you treat the life-threatening condition before all else. In outpatients, the patient with long-standing irritable bowel syndrome who is cachectic with a knobbly liver needs rapid investigation for malignant disease, and in general practice the woman who presents with a sore throat, mentions her chilblains and only later casually mentions a slightly lumpy neck needs to have her multinodular thyroid gland considered in some depth.

Share understanding

Share your findings with the patient

The reality is that this task usually comes immediately after the diagnostic/examination phase of the consultation. However involved they may be, the patient usually becomes passive and expectant while waiting for the revelatory pronouncements of the doctor. It is a skilful strategy to keep the patient involved, use their own words and continue to use the short-term memory of the previous exchanges. This explanation phase is the cornerstone of most consultations, and it often arises very quickly, even too quickly for many doctors.

Despite the difficulties, you must always try to explain your working diagnosis, what management options seem to be most appropriate and what the possible effects of any treatment are likely to be.

Tailor the explanation to the needs of the patient (sharing understanding)

By now you have got to know your patient a little. You should have a feel for the type of person they are, so that when you begin your explanation, you should ensure that your manner and language are appropriate to the patient's needs and that the information is presented in terms which they are likely to understand. A very common medical fault from the highest to the lowest is to cloud explanations with technical medical jargon that is incomprehensible to almost everyone. Don't do it.

Your explanation should be linked to the patient's beliefs, which you have already elicited. This does not mean that you have to adopt all of your patient's beliefs – some of them may be quite erroneous – but you must tailor your explanation to the unique human being who is sitting in front of you. This will make it much more relevant than the standard talk on hysterectomy or the routine explanation about irritable bowels. Consider the following examples.

- 'I know you are worried about the operation, particularly because Mum had such a bad time after her hysterectomy, but hers was for a different reason. You haven't got cancer like she had, and there is no reason for you to get depressed like your friend did. Has the surgeon explained what is going to be done?'

- 'This rash is called psoriasis, and it is caused by overactive cells in the skin, but it is probably not affected by what you eat' (having elicited the patient's belief that the rash was due to an allergy to certain foods).

- Another example is the common fear of a brain tumour in patients with headaches, and then tailoring the explanation to take this into account: 'I know you have been worried about brain tumour, but I think your other theory that it is migraine is correct, because . . .'

- 'I understand your concerns about the MMR vaccine. This is the best evidence we have, and there is no link with autism.'

- 'I know you are worried about becoming like your father who also had schizophrenia, but there are really effective treatments these days and you are a very different person.'

- 'You felt that the new tablets were to blame for these symptoms. That is possible, but if so the symptoms will wear off after a few weeks.'

- 'Although you feel that any activity makes the fatigue worse, research shows that gradually increasing activity actually helps.'

- 'You mentioned migraine and stress. I think stress is more likely because . . .'

Remember that an explanation is a one-way process, from doctor to patient, whereas a sharing of understanding is a two-way process and it cannot occur unless personal details, health understanding, concerns and expectations have been elicited in the first phase. Doctors who are sharing understanding are also formulating management plans and strategies while they are talking and listening. The act of sharing understanding is intended to clarify, modify and tailor the subsequent decision, making it more appropriate. Much of the effective sharing will be in the emotional realm of wants, needs, fears and irrational beliefs. Unemotional logic is not the stuff of most encounters. It is also important to realise that our patients' expectations of medicine's capacity to deliver diagnosis and cure will almost always outstrip the reality. This is a true understanding and not one in which most patients wish to share.

Ensure that the explanation is understood and accepted by the patient

Doctors, on balance, are quite good at giving explanations. The fly in the ointment is that patients are not good at understanding them. Watch your peers explaining to patients and ask yourself whether they are explaining for their patient's benefit or their own. Many explanations by doctors appear to be given in order to make the doctor feel that they have completed their own consulting process, and the patient is barely relevant. Ask yourself whether you are explaining for yourself or for your patient.

What you must do is to explain your understanding of what the nature of the problem is. At one end of the spectrum this may be too vague to be called an actual diagnosis, while at the other end it may be a clear-cut clinical entity. Even this is not enough – you must keep checking with your patient that they understand you. This is a process that requires considerable skill, and we shall touch on it again later, but be warned that a glassy-eyed, passive patient nodding obediently is not necessarily grasping every pearl of wisdom that falls from your lips. You must make some attempt to reconcile your viewpoint with that of your patient. What you are trying to achieve is a *shared understanding*, and this is different to a simple explanation. An explanation is a one-way process: 'I am the full vessel and I will pour my knowledge into the empty vessel that is my patient.' This does not work – it has to be a two-way process. Think instead of the patient as a melon seed who incorporates the water into their structure as they are growing.

Work from the MRCGP Consulting Skills module showed that checking our patients' understanding was the rarest of all observed behaviours, with less than 5% of doctors demonstrating it in three out of five selected consultations. This means that it must be difficult to do. So how can you make it easier? Here are a few suggestions.

- It clearly implies the use of a question; for example, 'Does that make sense?' or 'Have I made that clear?'
- Better still, try saying something like 'I know today's discussion has been complicated. Would you tell me what you are going to tell your partner about what we have said?' (Think of Mrs Arthur.)
- 'You may have found this difficult to understand. Would you like to tell me what you think we have agreed?'
- 'How would you explain your condition to someone else?'

- 'Is there anything you'd like to ask me?'
- 'What else do you want to know?'
- 'I don't know whether that makes sense?'

Some doctors ask patients, 'Can you just explain what I have just said back to me?' We think this is too direct and a rather paternalistic approach which makes patients feel exposed. 'Is that OK?' is just not good enough.

Share decisions and responsibility

Choose an appropriate form of management

Your management plan needs to be appropriate to your working diagnosis. This is part of the knowledge and skills taught at medical school and modified by experience throughout your career. Your management should of course reflect a good understanding of modern medical practice, and this is nowhere near as easy as it sounds. Medicine is ever changing, the slavish demands of evidence-based medicine weigh heavily, litigation lurks in every decision and pressure groups howl their demands from every corner. Uncertainty pervades all decisions. You can only do your best, and you have to keep working at that.

Involve the patient in the management plan to the appropriate extent

Patients should be involved in choosing their own management as much as possible, not least because their cooperation will be needed for the plan to be implemented. Management options should be shared with patients and, where appropriate, the patient should make the choice. This is another phase of explaining and sharing understanding, but this time it is about management, and the dialogue must be two-way. You may initially find this concept uncomfortable, but it is likely to make you more effective and less prone to 'medicalise'. Encouraging patients to see themselves as responsible for their own health may alter their locus of control a little and make them more likely to request information, as well as to use the medical profession more appropriately. As discussed previously, not all patients will want to be involved, and it is not always appropriate for them to be, but more often than not it is. If your patient is involved, the risk of litigation and disagreement is much lower. Try to work on this aspect of communication. It is a fairly rare behaviour in young registrars/trainees who are observed consulting.

Sharing decisions need not be too onerous. For example, consider a patient with tennis elbow. You could say something like 'Well, you've had it a few weeks now. I think the best thing is a cortisone injection – it's not too bad, you know. OK?' However, this is not sharing; it is telling. Alternatively, you could say, 'Well, you've tried the anti-inflammatory gel. I find physiotherapy works sometimes, or what about a splint for when you are working? They are often quite good. Or what do you think about a steroid injection?', to which the reply might be 'Er, well, doctor, what do you think would be best?' You might then say, 'Well, it is not necessarily an "either or" – the splint might be a good idea, but physio or the injection might be worth a try, too. Do you have a preference?' And so on. This is a dialogue.

Other examples of this approach include the following:
- 'So what do you feel about the strategies we have discussed?'
- 'Would you rather start the tablets now, or wait a few weeks and see if it settles?'
- 'I could refer you to our counsellor, or you could contact Relate yourself. Which would you prefer?'
- 'Some people prefer to adjust their dose (inhaler) themselves. If I give you some guidance, would you?'

The extent of the sharing will depend on the patient, how capable they are of engaging in such involvement, the nature of the problem, and what types of option exist.

Consider the following examples.
- A retired science teacher with newly diagnosed hypertension might expect (or need) to be involved very substantially in a variety of options, ranging from lifestyle modification, through choice of drugs, to the frequency and nature of follow-up.
- On the other hand, a learning-disabled teenager with severe tonsillitis might not appreciate a discussion of whether to take penicillin for 5 or 10 days! Here a simple consideration of whether to use tablets or liquid would be more appropriate (and more helpful).
- With a patient with tension headache you could discuss the treatments available, such as analgesics, relaxation techniques, referral for stress counselling, etc., and allow the patient to

indicate their preferred course of action. The patient with a sheaf of printouts of Internet articles about their condition demands a shared decision, and this situation is now commonplace.

How would you share options with Mrs Arthur?

The underlying idea is 'shared decision making', whether it is about medication, referral, investigations or taking time off work. However, it does have to be realistic. The doctor is the medical expert and the patient is the expert on himself or herself.

Make effective use of the consultation

Make efficient use of resources

Time

Perhaps the most precious resource of all is time. As King Richard II said, 'I wasted time, and now doth time waste me.' We must make efficient and sensible use of the available time and, if necessary, recommend further consultations as appropriate. The use of time by doctors is a subtle area of study. It is not the length that is so important, but the use to which the time is put. In general practice, it probably takes a minimum of eight well-used minutes to achieve a reasonable degree of shared management and shared understanding. It probably takes longer in outpatients, as the doctor usually does not know the patient at all. There have been many studies on time spent with patients in all kinds of settings, and the interesting fact that emerges is that the amount of time spent does not seem to affect patient satisfaction significantly. This fact should remind us that it is the use to which we put the time that matters. Some doctors can waffle away for 15 minutes with no difficulty, while others can be patient-focused, enquiring and efficient within half of that timescale.

'To consult well takes time – this is now unarguable' stated Professor George Freeman and colleagues in their *British Medical Journal* article (Freeman *et al.*, 2002), although we could argue with this just a bit. As we have said, a good consulter will do more with the time than a poor one, and many can achieve in 10 minutes what a disorganised consulter has not achieved in 20. This is of course too subtle for most research. One quality marker has been that longer consultations contain more health promotion – well, hallelujah, but just a small dose of caution here. When the MRCGP examination piloted the consulting skills criteria, we found health promotion by doctors to be a destructive process in many, if not most, cases. To trained GP observers the doctor's agenda effectively swamped that of the patient. You may find it worrying that in order to earn more money GPs need to practise this skill daily – thus more and more time given over to a quality-standard agenda and less and less time for what the patient actually came about. This, of course, may ultimately be good for the health of the nation, although not for that of its Exchequer. Time will tell, but not in our lifetime we suspect. Will it be of any benefit for Mrs Arthur?

Increasingly, other health professionals are the first port of call for patients, and if not then most of the work of doctors is in multi-disciplinary teams these days. Patients are likely to see a community psychiatric nurse (CPN) before the psychiatrist in clinic, or the nurse practitioner for triage before the dermatologist. Other health professionals may refer to you. Sometimes this may be entirely appropriate. Other times this may reflect a profound misunderstanding of what you perceive to be your role.

Investigations

Any investigations that you order should be capable of confirming or excluding the working diagnosis. There should be no place for arm-fuls of blood to satisfy every whim of the overzealous higher trainee. Costs are important and should be justified in terms of the refinements that any results might make to the overall management of the patient. If a test will not make any difference to the outcome or the management of any particular case, it will be very hard to justify. Always ask yourself, 'Why am I doing this test? Will it clarify, confirm or refute what I suspect? Is it really necessary? Am I doing it just to reassure?'

We often do tests just to reassure our patients that there is nothing wrong, but unless their true fears are addressed, diagnostic tests may leave them more anxious than they were before. Several recent studies have confirmed this truism. The usual culprit in cases of failure to reassure is poor communication. A survey of 5150 patients who had recently been discharged from hospital revealed that 34% of them had not been told the results of tests. In a study conducted by cardiologists in Melbourne in 1996, it was found that many patients continued to be anxious about their heart despite being informed of a normal echocardiography result. Furthermore, three-quarters of the patients in this sample were referred for exclusion of heart disease after routine examination for insurance or employment purposes, which suggests that unjustified concern about ill health is often iatrogenic. Thus it is clear that informing patients about a normal diagnostic result may not always succeed in reassuring them. Ambiguous or false-positive results may create or worsen anxiety. It is much better to get your patient's fears out into the open than to perform unnecessary further tests or make an unnecessary specialist referral.

Other (health) professionals

You must consider the possible involvement of other professionals, such as nurses, physiotherapists or other medical specialists. Only make referrals when these are necessary and appropriate as decided in your agreed management plan with the patient.

Prescribing

The cost of drugs is forever escalating, and the burden on national resources caused by inappropriate, uneconomical and unused drugs is enormous. Whenever you prescribe, ask yourself the following questions:

- Is a prescription really necessary?
- Is this the best choice of drug(s) for the condition?
- Could I obtain the same efficacy more economically?
- Will my patient take the drug(s)?

This last question is relevant in several ways. We have already discussed some issues relating to concordance. Another issue concerns our patients' understanding of the tablets that they are prescribed. Side-effect leaflets are now included in all packs, but are couched in such bald and frightening terms that many of our patients read these leaflets, become afraid and then angry, don't take the drugs, and then storm in to see us demanding to know why we prescribed such a potentially lethal drug as ibuprofen. There is convincing observational evidence that doctors do not discuss the pros and cons of various prescribed drugs very often – at best it is peremptory. This is another area that we shall all really have to work on with regard to our communication with our patients. We must take steps to improve prescribing concordance and, as you are now aware, this means seeking out our patient's understanding of the treatment and a reactive explanation based on that understanding. Explaining side effects and the concepts of cost and benefit and relative risk is immensely difficult, but we have to do it, and with practice we can only get better.

Research in the area of prescribing can be worrying. Here are a few examples of the results of recent respectable studies.

- When the doctor thinks that the patient expects a prescription, they are 10 times more likely to prescribe.
- Patients who expect a prescription are three times more likely to receive one as those who do not.
- Prescribing antibiotics for sore throats has only a marginal effect on the resolution of symptoms, but enhances the belief in antibiotics and intention to consult in future when compared with strategies of non- or delayed prescribing.
- Shared decision making about drugs is very unusual.
- Patient satisfaction with non-prescribing is related to the resolution of their concerns.
- Doctors rarely discuss side effects in detail.
- Major misunderstandings related to prescribing are common, and are due to patients not being able to voice their agenda about their health understanding.
- In cases of atrial fibrillation, taking account of patient preferences would lead to far fewer prescriptions for anticoagulants than under published guideline recommendations.

And there is some recent good news for this seventh edition:

- Enhanced communication skills significantly reduce antibiotic prescribing for lower respiratory tract infections without compromising patient recovery and satisfaction with care.
- These skills involved exploring ideas, concerns and expectations (ICE), sharing and then checking patient understanding.
- Exploring ICE leads to a reduction in the number of new prescriptions.

Establish an effective relationship with the patient

The word 'effective' is the crux here. What you wish to achieve is a relationship that helps you to complete the other tasks. You must discover the reasons for the patient's attendance, define the clinical problem, address the patient's problem, explain effectively, attempt to share some of the decision making, and make overall effective use of the consultation. How you achieve this is your business. You may well have been taught interpersonal skills such as empathising, eye contact, use of touch, and so on. These are all very well, but if used unthinkingly they may simply produce clones of slightly damp Methodist ministers who are just too warm and hold your hand for five seconds too long (apologies to Methodists, but we had to upset someone). We have all met lovely, warm, empathetic doctors who are frankly ineffective, and we have also come across some pretty unpleasant cold fish who are at least efficient, though never really effective because of their deficient communication. It almost does not matter whether you consult in green spotted pyjamas wearing a goofy hat if you can regularly achieve a shared management plan and a shared understanding. It is the achievement that matters, not the means of getting there.

We are exaggerating, but not a lot. There are, of course, some styles of behaviour that are more likely to produce an effective relationship than others, not least a genuine expression of interest in your patient as a fellow human being, but there is no one style that will suit all. In longer-term relationships it may be the building up of mutual respect leading to trust that is crucial in a therapeutic sense. Even with trust there are problems, as a very trusting patient may stop participating.

Concentrate on your strengths and what you feel comfortable with, and work on your effectiveness. If you are consistently failing to achieve an effective relationship with patients, some of the analytical methods discussed later in this book may help you to diagnose your problem and find an appropriate remedy.

Give opportunistic health promotion advice

There are some areas of preventive behaviour about which we as a profession are pretty convinced; for example, smoking is bad for you, immunisation is good for you, as is regular moderate exercise, and probably regular cervical smears, etc. Other dietary and lifestyle messages depend on your beliefs, such as the value of regular breast self-examination, cholesterol watching, egg eating and salmonella, and the legions of other advice in the 'Nanny knows best' style. You have to make the best decisions you can on the basis of the available evidence. The point at issue here is whether you should take an appropriate moment in the consultation to give such advice. Linking lifestyle advice to a current illness can be quite an effective way of altering behaviour. Just telling patients to stop smoking and giving them a leaflet will mean that 5%–10% will give up – an astonishingly high figure when you think of how many patients you see. This is where motivational interviewing (MI) styles work well. Short consultations which explore patients understanding of their problem behaviour and help them weigh up the factors for and against changing it are much more effective than repeating to them that their behaviour is dangerous. MI helps people move into the action phase of the contemplation cycle mentioned earlier.

This is another area for you to think about. The consultation does provide the opportunity for such advice, but not to the exclusion of the patient's agenda. Butler and colleagues reported in the *British Medical Journal* in 1998 that repeatedly advising patients to stop smoking was likely to be ineffective, even counter-productive. They showed that intervention was much more likely to be effective if it was patient-centred and respectful of individuals' circumstances, attitudes and choices.

As we have already intimated in the section on time, it has become clear in the last two decades that this task, now an integral part of every GP's contract, has grave implications for effective communication if it is misused. It is very obvious that it needs to be performed sensitively and in the context of the patient's stated or implied wishes, and it must not be allowed to obscure the patient's agenda.

Examples of what *not* to do include the following:
- 'Let's leave your headaches and talk about your cholesterol.'
- 'Here's a tissue – now when is your next mammogram?'
- 'The computer says you are here for your BP check, so up with the sleeve.'
- 'I think smoking is more important to discuss than your legs, don't you?'

Safety netting

At the end of the consultation you must set the appropriate conditions and the timescale for your patient to return for review, in terms of their symptoms or some other parameter; for example, a falling peak flow reading. Even the worst management plan in the world can be rescued with an effective safety net. Unfortunately, many missed opportunities and complaints arise from a failure of doctors to do this.

Shared decision making: a recap

In the twenty-first century the goal of most consultations must be to achieve a level of shared decision making. Let us go through the necessary elements again. Truly shared decision making requires a partnership with your patient. You must establish your patient's preference with regard to the amount and type of information and clarify their wish for involvement. You must also respond to their ideas, concerns and expectations. It is now that you must seek to achieve a shared understanding and allow your patient to reflect upon and assess the impact of alternative decisions with regard to their values and lifestyle. You must share the management options, identify choices and, if necessary, evaluate the research evidence in relation to the individual patient. To complete the task you must negotiate and finally agree upon an action plan, and if necessary make arrangements for follow-up. This added burden on the modern doctor is onerous but, if done properly, hopefully enjoyable and satisfying.

We must emphasise again that this goal of effective, sharing communication does not come easily. It is not a natural human style – it really has to be practised in order to be learnt. But it is worth the effort.

With regard to what you wish to achieve with your patients as the years go by, here are a couple of poems to get you thinking. The first is by WH Auden, and was his description of the type of doctor he wanted for himself.

> Give me a doctor partridge plump,
> short in the leg and broad in the rump,
> an endomorph with gentle hands,
> who'll never make absurd demands
> that I abandon all my vices,
> or pull a long face in a crisis,
> but with a twinkle in his eye
> will tell me that I have to die.

The second poem, by Marie Campkin, is a chilling updated version.

> Give me a doctor underweight,
> Computerised and up to date.
> A businessman who understands
> accountancy and target bands.
> Who demonstrates sincere devotion
> to audit and to health promotion –
> but when my outlook's for the worse
> refers me to the practice nurse.

References

Barry CA, Bradley CP, Britten N *et al.* Patients' unvoiced agendas in general practice consultations: qualitative study. *BMJ.* 2000; **320**: 1246–50.

Butler CC, Pill R, Stott NC. Qualitative study of patients' perceptions of doctors' advice to quit smoking: implications for opportunistic health promotion. *BMJ.* 1998; **316**(7148): 1878–81.

Freeman GK, Horder JP, Howie JGR *et al.* Evolving general practice consultation in Britain: issues of length and context. *BMJ.* 2002; **324**(7342): 880–2.

CHAPTER 7

Ways of looking at your own communication

- You have to want to improve.
- To improve you have to watch yourself interacting with patients.
- To learn from this you need constructive feedback.
- It is worth it, honestly!

The first problem with looking at your own communication with your patients is that you have to *want* to do it, but nobody wants to look at their inept, stumbling and wooden performances, do they? Why wear a hair shirt unless you are a monk? Life is just too short. No! We can't let you get away with that sort of defensive thinking. You owe it to your patients and, what is more, if you learn to look properly you will find it fascinating, illuminating and immensely rewarding.

Creating a climate for learning

What you wish to achieve is a climate for achieving true constructive formative feedback on your patient communication strengths and weaknesses. Looking at yourself consulting is unnerving initially. Others looking at you can be terrifying. Why is this? There are several reasons. There is the fear of being found wanting, of being exposed, and of being attacked and ridiculed. There are certain taboos in our society about what one cannot criticise, car driving and lovemaking being the two most obvious examples. For doctors, talking to their patients could be a third.

Our medical school training often does not help – most of us are used to a point-scoring, adversarial, one-upmanship style of teaching. You have to know one more syndrome than your colleague, think of the blood test no one else has thought of, and take pretty fierce criticism on the chin. Some years ago, a nervous young student was having the mysteries of a diabetic retinitis demonstrated by an aggressive and impatient chief. The student had not fully grasped the skills of ophthalmoscopy, but he was desperately trying to maintain some personal credibility with his irascible tutor. 'Well, what do you see?' To all observing, including the chief, the ophthalmoscope light was now brightly illuminating a patch of pillow to the left of the patient's head, and it was obvious that the young man was not seeing anything of the retina. Gamely, but unwisely, he continued to give a fictitious description of what he was not yet skilled enough to see. The chief bellowed at him, 'You silly little worm – if you had an IQ of one less you would be a plant.' This form of unconstructive feedback is not likely to make us keen to reveal our innermost secrets to a group of doctors and will certainly not be formative in any useful way. So how can we create a protected environment? It's easy – there are just two rules.

Rules for formative feedback on doctor–patient interactions

- Rule 1. Good points first.
- Rule 2. No criticism without recommendation.

There you are – simple, eh? There is actually a third rule, which is *always obey the first two*.

Simple these rules might be, but that does not mean they are always easy to keep and enforce. Let us look at rule 1 first and imagine you are working in a little study group preparing for PACES, MRCS, FCEM, MRCGP exams etc. You have either role played a scenario or shown an actual recording of a patient interview of yours. Your colleague starts the ball rolling with: 'Great. OK, now what did you do well?' If you are not prepared for this question you might easily demonstrate the 'goldfish sign'. A glazed look spreads over your physiognomy, your mouth begins to open and shut involuntarily but emits no sound, and your confusion has stymied your thinking. This is because you are not used to recognising what you did well. In all probability you have been watching yourself with mounting self-disgust.

> Oh Lord, look at that, I missed that cue altogether. Gosh, I am glad
> my professor didn't see that examination. What a rotten explanation.
> I don't think I understood it, let alone the patient. She will never come
> back. I was just so awful . . . and then some wally asks what I did
> well! I didn't do anything well! It was all terrible! Oh God . . .

Ah, but you did. You did many things very well indeed. You may need a little practice to recognise your strengths, but recognise them you must or the baby goes out with the bath water. Learning from watching yourself interact with patients must be a building exercise, not a destruction exercise.

If you are watching with a colleague or a teacher, it seems to work best if you start the discussion. In other words, the doctor being observed should start any discussion with what they did well. It is often necessary to clear away matters of fact, but don't be side-tracked into covert criticism. 'Which drug did you prescribe?' is fine, but 'Do you normally examine the chest through the shirt?' is not. If you are having difficulty recognising your strengths, this is when your colleague or teacher can help. No criticisms should be made at all at this stage. Only when you have a thorough understanding of what you did well and the skills you used to achieve your strengths should you move on to areas where you think you were less effective.

Doctors are very good at being critical. After all, we are not stupid. The problem is that our talent for supportive, formative and constructive criticism is often underdeveloped. There is no place for criticism without recommendation.

> Liz, I thought when you asked her if she was worried about cancer
> and she began to cry, that you might have helped her more and per-
> haps discovered a little more of her fear. If you had just let her cry
> for a few moments, maybe asked her why she was crying instead of
> just carrying on a little abruptly. I wonder if you were afraid of the
> emotions she might release?

This is fine. You may not agree with all of the comments, but you have been given some positive suggestions about your behaviour which you can use or not, and the discussion can be an open but sensitive one in which you are not unduly threatened.

> Liz, you were a bit insensitive when she started to cry. You must work on that and do better next time.

This is unhelpful because you do not know what to work on and you are just left feeling vaguely inadequate.

A problem has arisen in some groups that use 'good points first' rules, in that a degree of cynicism develops. Over the years two useful terms have been coined that highlight this difficulty. These are the 'Blodgit', which is the standard unit of insincere praise, and the 'Shit Sandwich', which indicates that if you are not careful everything before the 'but what could you have done better?' question is bullshit. Only integrity, honesty and practice can get rid of this, otherwise the exercise will degenerate into a sham.

Start using the rules now with your friends, and try to persuade some of your teachers to follow suit. In our experience of groups there is sometimes initial frustration at the constraints imposed by these rules, and someone will inevitably say: 'Come on, Liz, stop pussyfooting about. Hit me with what you really think. What am I bad at?'

The trouble with this approach is that eventually the teacher can relent and do just what has been requested. The result is obvious in the metaphorical sense. If you hit a human being hard enough they will always fall over, and that is what happens, and why the rules are there in the first place. Don't break them. Using such rules does not mean that you cannot touch on difficult personal areas and areas of special sensitivity. It just means that it takes time to create a supportive, trusting environment in which such delicate and meaningful discussions can genuinely take place to the considerable benefit of the learner, namely you.

Ways of looking

You do not need high-tech equipment to look at you interacting with a patient. For a start, thinking over what you have just achieved with a patient is useful. Being observed by a colleague who can give you supportive formative feedback helps, and all that needs is an extra chair. Psychotherapy departments are prone to one-way mirrors, although we must confess to never feeling comfortable with such a set-up. The disadvantage of all of those methods is that there is no action replay. The advantage is that patient consent, although it should always be asked for, does not need to be formalised.

Real patients

On balance, most people do not mind being observed, discussed or recorded, but there have to be rules and respect for the individual. Patients know when they go to hospitals that they will be seen more often than not by at least two doctors, and often by a pack of them. This is no excuse at all for the time-honoured medical practice of then discussing a fellow human being as if they were an antique clock, with the occasional excruciatingly patronising aside.

> 'Have you noticed how pale she is? Haemoglobin probably about 6. The myelodysplasia is obviously progressing. Have you noticed her nails are clubbing? Fascinating, really.'
>
> Turning casually to patient: 'Don't worry, nothing that a little top up with red cells can't fix.'

Patients should be involved as much as possible in discussions about their condition. Detailed, jargon-ridden speculation should be continued outside their hearing. If any form of recording of the interview is to be made, the patient's written permission should be sought. The patient should opt in, not out, and have an opportunity to opt out afterwards. Visual and audio recordings should be erased after the teaching session, and if they are required for a larger presentation, the patient's written permission should be sought again, preferably after allowing him or her to see or hear the recording.

Sadly, the rules around information governance and the Data Protection Act seem impenetrably complicated these days. Any information with patient information on it is supposed to be securely stored on encrypted data sticks or devices with passwords. They are meant to be securely transported in locked boxes and kept locked in clinical areas. Consent can overcome much of this, but it is certainly off-putting to doctors new to the arena and a barrier to using this helpful form of communication training. There are few experienced doctors outside primary care who can offer constructive feedback on this at present. Maybe you can help change this?

Patients are less passive in the less frightening and more familiar general practice setting, and are more likely to assert themselves by refusing permission to be observed. There have been many studies on refusal rates (which range from 1% to 60%), and the variables that seem to be most important (other than the patient) are the ambience of the practice and the way in which the message is sold. A gruff receptionist telling a new patient that 'Dr Tate is filming tonight, but you don't have to have it' is likely to elicit a much higher refusal rate than a patient who has been told when she booked an appointment that the surgery is being recorded for internal teaching purposes, especially if she is given a leaflet on arrival offering further explanation, including assurance that any personal examination will not be on camera. Curiously, the actual condition, including problems with naughty bits, etc., does not consistently explain patients' refusal. It is better to sort out permission outside the consulting room in order to ensure that the dynamics are not upset too much.

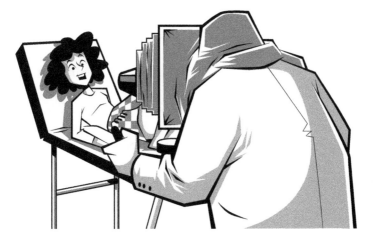

Patients do not worry unduly about being observed, and it does not change their behaviour in any significant way. Two decades ago, a younger Peter had a moderately conspicuous camera *in situ* for several months – always switched off, of course – without explicit permission, and only one person commented on it in all that time. This was a young woman requiring an internal examination who, while in a compromising position, suddenly spotted the camera and said demurely, 'Do I smile now?'

The two methods of recording that are currently in use are digital audio and camcorders (either DVD or hard disc). Videotape and audiotape are nearly extinct. Audio recording is cheap, unobtrusive and easy, but pretty boring. Visual recording is much more stimulating – you catch the expressions and the non-verbal behaviour, and it is just more likely to hold your attention. However, it is more complicated, more difficult to set up, more threatening and more can go wrong. Having said all that, almost all families have now used a camcorder at some stage, they will certainly have used a mobile phone, and the technology is pretty familiar. Modern equipment is sensitive to low light, so will work in the dingiest of outpatient suites or surgeries. It is all colour these days, and all new equipment will date and (more usefully) time stamp the recording. There are still a variety of formats, which can be confusing. The smaller, more convenient camcorders are rapidly becoming solid state, and allow easy transfer to DVD or memory stick. This is ideal for building a portfolio of consultations, assuming you have the requisite permission, and such equipment is becoming quite cheap.

The on-camera microphones are now quite good, but if you want better sound quality (and it is poor sound quality that ruins more recordings than anything else) you should use an external microphone. Many hospitals have audiovisual departments that can help, and all general practice trainers these days have experience of regular recording. Many general practices now have fixed camera brackets in surgeries, but most will need a tripod. A wide-angle lens is very helpful, as many consulting areas are fairly cramped. Although you can simply double the focal length by bouncing off a mirror, you will lose light. However, modern cameras are so light sensitive that this does not matter. The aim must be to have both patient and doctor in shot with clear facial expressions. If you can only get one clearly, go for the patient.

Being observed by a colleague

All hospital doctors do this all the time, but how many of them utilise this as a tool for improving their communication? However, workplace-based assessments (WPBA) ensure that all doctors in training have to be observed talking to patients by senior colleagues at least sometimes. The feedback is supposed to be formative, although in many cases it is still treated as a test to be passed or failed and little meaningful learning takes place. Emphasis in hospital inevitably falls on the content of the interaction (correct diagnosis and management) rather than the process. To improve your communication skills you will have to find a like-minded colleague or trainer. If you are really stuck find a good course in your area or buy some communication-teaching DVDs.

Simulated patients

Since the first edition of this book was published in 1994, there has been an explosion in the simulated patient industry. All postgraduate exams involve simulated patients these days as do most training courses. Every major hospital has a simulation centre and a huge bank of actors who portray every known human condition with startling accuracy.

We have some caveats, but on balance this is not a bad thing, and if you ever get the opportunity to work with actors or health professionals simulating real patients, do take it. You can obtain really useful feedback from an articulate, non-passive patient telling you what they really thought about your strengths and your less effective strategies. The wonderful thing about simulation as a learning tool is the fact that in real life it is almost impossible to know what any patient's 'script' is. In simulation this is known, so you can see how far you got.

Simulation is also very useful for short-circuiting your learning circle, as it is able to produce particular patients with particular problems on demand. The next assessment development is likely to be the simulated real patient – if you see what we mean – turning up in your surgery/outpatients pretending to be a newly diagnosed diabetic. This technique has demonstrated with stark clarity that doctors do not do in real life what they say they will do in examinations.

There is a commonly quoted pyramid of the assessment of clinical competence (Miller's), which includes communication (*see* Figure 7.1).

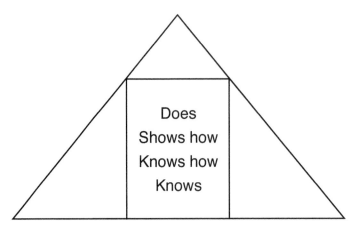

FIGURE 7.1 Miller's pyramid for the assessment of clinical competence

Direct observation is at the top, simulation is 'Shows how', and knowing is a long way from doing. Just stop and reflect for a minute or two on the implications of this pyramid.

For many doctors in higher training the consulting element is tested by simulation. This is efficient, repeatable and (very) expensive, but what worries us is the encouragement of fast checklist behaviour to the exclusion of true curiosity about the human being in front of you. You can't simulate curiosity – it simply becomes hollow acting and little else. So learn how to consult to pass your exams, but please learn to consult properly as well.

While writing this edition a furore has developed regarding discriminatory pass rates in simulated communication exams, particularly the MRCGP. We do not pretend to have the answer to this worrying development but suggest that some cultures may adapt better than others to simulated interactions, including such highly rated skills as empathy, compassion and curiosity. It may be that on occasions we are marking acting ability as opposed to actual performance. All the more reason to try very hard to improve you own performance with real patients not just pretend ones.

Role play

Role play is do-it-yourself simulation and it can be very useful. Unfortunately, most people come out in a rash as soon as it is mentioned and cannot be found for days. It has always seemed to us that this fear is misplaced because, so long as the rules are strictly enforced, role play has some safety valves built into it. The first of these is that it is artificial, and that is a legitimate defence for erratic performance, especially early on. The second is that we all vary in our ability to act, and being a terrible actor is not synonymous with poor medicine – the opposite also applies. The enormous strength of role play is the occasion when you play the patient. Here you can really put yourself into their role and begin to understand what it feels like. This is worth much embarrassment and angst, and you really must seize every opportunity you get, as it truly will make you a better doctor. Another advantage of role play is that it requires no technology, although a recording does improve its usefulness.

CHAPTER 8

Attitude – the magic move?

- Too much thinking can make us stupid.
- Remember it is what matters to the patient that really counts.

We have had a change of heart in the last few years and now believe that most doctor–patient skills come naturally, but that the attitudes and the confidence do not. You will have heard sports coaches urge pupils to visualise the perfect serve or drive and then let their instincts take over, so it will by now be clear to you that the first step is to think about what you wish to achieve (we did this in Chapter 6). But that is not enough, so in this chapter we shall consider whether we really do want to do it properly. If so, we must learn to communicate intelligently, but is there also a 'magic move' to help us jump from the ordinary to the excellent?

We suspect that you have occasionally mused on the confusing evolutionary merits of intelligence. We have found no fossil trilobites with large brains – and they were around for aeons of geological time. Then the amazingly big dinosaurs ate, fought and farted around (literally) for a huge time span without ever finding the need to develop mobile phones. So why in the last few seconds of geological time have we evolved intelligence?

Looked at dispassionately, our intelligence has not been an unmitigated success. We can destroy ourselves on a scale undreamed of in the animal kingdom, and with our capacity to meddle on a large scale we can now destabilise our planet even more quickly than the vagaries of the cosmic forces that surround us. Human scientific progress is now being made at a speed so fast that it makes no sense when compared with the relatively slow pace of evolution, even in human history. After all, since 'intelligence' arrived on the scene, progress has certainly not been relentless. Those wonderful and esoteric Egyptians came from nowhere to instant technological wizardry. The Great Pyramid is still literally unbelievable, the second one is impressive but not as good, and in no time they couldn't build them at all. They could still mould Tutankhamen's awe-inspiring funerary mask 1000 years later, but they carried on 'going backwards' slowly for another 1000 years until Cleopatra finished it off for good.

Ah, we hear you say, but what has all of this to do with communication? Well, we are going to argue that by trying to be clever we forget our instincts. The real problem is that we are not clever enough – our much vaunted intelligence is pretty superficial, and to understand things at all we have to reduce complexities to simple building blocks, thus distorting the true nature of the phenomenon. The number of blocks gets nowhere near the mystery of the Great Pyramid. An equation cannot describe the beauty or the mind-numbing infiniteness of a Mandelbrot fractal, and a deep understanding of the Krebs cycle doesn't help most doctors to cure anyone. Added to this, we become ridiculously possessive and overbearing about the small pieces of knowledge that we have gleaned. Consider the health professions. Cholesterol is bad for you, as is too much fat. Smoking is anathema and obesity is a dangerous state. All such statements have some truth in them but take no account of values, human instinct or experience, and the real truth is much more complex and multivariate, and capable of being viewed from many different perspectives. Health messages become reduced to little more than slogans, and the complex instinctive nature of human decision making is not acknowledged. We have evolved to make decisions about situations and our fellow human beings almost instantly. Remember system 1 and system 2. For example, we are often attracted to another person across a crowded room, and sometimes we dislike someone on sight. We know from personal experience that our original impressions are mostly but not always confirmed. Human conversation is based on previous experience, unconscious observations, pheromones, feelings and hunches, but most of our interacting with patients is not, although it should be.

We all learn how to communicate from a very early age, and most of us are not taught in the conventional sense. When our teachers do attack us with subjunctives, gerunds, past participles and split infinitives (and tell us we can't boldly go), some of us are instinctively irritated, some of us make it a lifetime study, and most just put such grammatical pontifications to the back of our minds to be remembered in exams and interviews, but not important in our daily existence.

The point is that we are creatures with only a modicum of intelligence, but we do carry with us a barrel-load of attitudes. What is an attitude? The *Oxford English Dictionary* says that it is a considered and permanent disposition or reaction to a person or thing. You might quibble with 'considered', as many of the attitudes that you have are not considered we suspect; they just are – visceral, instinctive and sometimes clearly tribal. Some of them you will not be proud of, so you won't tell anyone what they are, and probably, like us, spend a lot of your life hiding some of these attitudes lest you end up with few friends. Most human prejudices are attitudes, too. Attitudes are only very loosely related to intelligence. They tend to come from the midbrain, not the cortex, and they are based on survival instincts and emotional feedback loops that are difficult to dissect and often not amenable to logical understanding.

The point we wish to make about attitudes is that they govern our behaviour. Your heart may sink at this juncture and you may stop reading because this point is so obvious – all that for this! But if you will bear with us we would just like to point out that most conventional educational theory implies, and in some cases even states, that *knowledge* governs behaviour. The health educators are driven unceasingly (and fruitlessly) by this belief. We are not saying that knowledge does not influence behaviour, but it only works when what is learned changes an *attitude* about, say, a procedure, a screening opportunity or a loosely held belief (e.g. for or against the legalisation of cannabis). This of course makes the point that not all attitudes are equal – some are much more entrenched than others and much less amenable to the voice of sweet reason. Here again we must disagree with the *Oxford English Dictionary*'s use of the word 'permanent', as attitudes do change, but usually slowly. Now if we doctors concentrated on finding out the attitudes of our patients to the slings and arrows of outrageous medicine, we might be more effective in steering them towards doing what is currently thought to be good for them.

Of course, the same applies to us – we have attitudes, too. When our own attitudes clash with those of our patients, we can only rely on 'professionalism' to help us through, followed by a strong cup of coffee and a gripe to our colleagues. Trying to find out what our patients' attitudes are implies that we are minded to do so – in other words, we have an attitude to an attitude.

People's attitudes are not necessarily what they say they are. This again is not a revelation but an uneasy truth about a common lie. In most medical viva examinations examiners are taught not just to expose the attitudes of the candidate (e.g. for or against termination), but also to seek their justification of that attitude, the argument being that you can't really mark attitudes out of 10, but you can have a stab at rank ordering the justifications. This is not easy, and one person's justification is another's bigotry. Justifications tend of course to be post-hoc cortical intellectualisations of inherently midbrain feelings. Exam candidates, almost without exception, claim that they believe in and practise the patient-centred method, and most, particularly in primary care and psychiatry, can describe several consulting models and the concepts behind them to the satisfaction of the examiners. However, when video recordings of actual interactions are scrutinised, only 10% can demonstrate actually doing it regularly in encounters which they had selected to demonstrate just that method. Here there is a breakdown in the theory – the stated attitudes do not lead to the stated behaviour, so the attitude must not be the real one, and the candidates are not telling the truth (remember the pyramid in Chapter 7). Are you one of them? Why do you find it so hard to do? Think about it now – put the book down, and think about your attitudes to patients and communicating. This is the 'magic move' – it is all to do with your real attitude.

Practising patient-centred medicine is in fact pretty easy if you want to do it – you just have to listen, be curious and participate in a dialogue rather than a monologue, but you do have to *want* to do it. Ask yourself, do I really want to involve my patients? If not, why not?

Communication courses have for years used models of educational behaviour – tasks, strategies and skills abound. There have been many programmes full of skilful simulated patients, hours of dissecting videotapes, and clever skills-training workshops, some even run by Peter the elder author! But, and it is a very big but, the changes in actual doctor behaviour have been agonisingly slow. Again, why is this? The simple answer is that the majority of the profession still do not regard patient-centred, evidence-based, shared decision making as worth the time and emotional effort to them, and if they feel like that, all of the knowledgeable and clever teaching in the world is going to make very little, if any, difference. Is that how you feel?

In fact, the majority of humans, as we have previously intimated, do not need much teaching in communication. In our personal experience, many young registrars have become really 'good' communicators almost overnight in the sense of involving their patients, following a real attitude change brought about by an overbearing trainer or a realisation of the annoying consequences of failing the impending postgraduate examination. Of course they can then improve, and practise the skills until they become automatic and instinctive, but the first and fundamental step is the change in attitude. If we think about our attitudes, our intelligence might be useful. Get the attitude right by thinking, then let instinct, experience and evolution take over and the results are almost magical. John Lennon was wrong – all you need is attitude, but it has to be the right one, and there is the rub. So the first step towards improving your communication skills is to get your attitude right. Keep thinking about it.

Good therapeutic interaction with your patients need not be difficult or shrouded in mystery. We suggest that you make a list such as the following 14 questions and pin it up in front of you. Let us highlight the second and fourth questions, about curiosity and what matters. If you are curious, it means that you want to know more – about your patient, their illness and their feelings. What matters to patients is the important part of their health understanding – a mixture of ideas, concerns, expectations and the reasons for coming to see you. The first time you can answer 'yes' to all 14 questions, give yourself a pat on the back or, better still, a special treat. The second time you do it, you can allow yourself a small sense of triumph, and by the third time you will know that you can communicate effectively.

Questions to ask yourself after the interaction

1 Do I know significantly more about this patient than I did before they came in through the door?
2 Was I curious?
3 Did I really listen?
4 Did I find out what really mattered to them?
5 Did I explore their agenda, including their beliefs and expectations?
6 Did I make an acceptable working diagnosis?

7 Did I use what they thought when I started explaining?
8 Did I give them the opportunity to be involved in decisions?
9 Did I explore their understanding of the treatment?
10 Did I make some attempt to check that they really understood?
11 Did we agree on (1) the diagnosis, (2) the management and (3) the follow-up?
12 Have I recorded the salient information?
13 Was I friendly?
14 Did I do this in an appropriate timescale?

Now a plea to teachers in medical schools, hospitals and primary care. 'History taking' is Victorian, patronising and, in most hands, communicatively disastrous. In an attempt to keep it simple, we only ask that every time a student or young doctor is asked to recite 'the history', the first questions are the following:

- What is the patient concerned about?
- What do they expect?
- What really matters to them?

Spotting real empathy

Now let us go bird-watching. There are two species on which we would like you to become experts, so that you can tell them apart at a glance – but we warn you, it will take practice.

The first bird is the 'common nice mumble'. This is what many of us mean when we pretend to be patient-centred. It looks like this.

Hello, Mrs Arthur, I bet the traffic was awful . . . Don't worry about the thyroid gland, we will get it sorted for you . . . are you having a holiday this year? [while filling in a blood test form] . . . I bet your husband is worried about you [still filling in the form, and paying no attention to her response] . . . Well, now, off you go and get these tests done – we will see you with the results soon and then fix the right treatment for you. It has been really nice to meet you, and you mustn't worry about anything.

The second bird is much, much rarer and is known as the 'lesser spotted empathy'. Here is an example of a young one – not in full plumage yet, but one day it could turn into a fine specimen.

Hello, Mrs Arthur, you have finally made it to outpatients, so what has been on your mind? . . . Is that what you were worried about? Cancer like your aunt? I hope not, but you are in the right place for us to make the correct diagnosis and give you the right treatment . . . What do you know about the thyroid gland? . . . We may have to give you some radiation treatment with a special iodine. How do you feel about that? . . . I don't think that is a risk to you getting pregnant, but I will find out more details from my registrar and get back to you, plus the hospital leaflet to read. Next time we can go through some of your worries . . . There are those options we talked about – what thoughts have you got? . . . What are you going to tell your husband about what we have talked about? . . . No, no, that's not right, you won't need an operation at present because as I explained . . . See you in a month, hope you have a good holiday. Bye.

The common nice mumble is a robust bird, like the cuckoo, and can easily push the more delicate lesser spotted empathy out of the nest. The lesser spotted empathy also takes longer to learn to fly, with many abortive attempts and much flapping, and in its youth it can be a rather bedraggled, disillusioned-looking creature. But in maturity it is a beauty to behold. It is our fervent hope that as we improve the environment, this species will at last flourish and become the dominant one, but there is a long way to go.

In 2008, a US study identified a hardening of heart among medical students during their years at medical school, as they steadily lost the empathy with which they had started. Thus they started their careers on the caring back foot, as it were, and it will take a real effort for them to recover.

Let us finish with a few words on how to recognise the lesser spotted empathy. Empathy, as defined by the *Oxford English Dictionary*, is the power of identifying oneself with, and so fully comprehending, the person who is the subject of contemplation. How can doctors attempt to do this without eliciting their patients' ideas, concerns and expectations? And does it matter? Oh yes it does. In an impassioned essay on the importance of empathy published in the *British Medical Journal* in 2005, Dr Craig Watson, an Aberdeenshire GP, finished with the following paragraph:

> In this age of science and technology and rapid access to limitless information, our powerful computers seem unable to calculate the value of what really matters. In defending the role, status, income and future of community doctors, science and statistics will no doubt play their part. However, because they form only part of our work they should also form only part of the debate. I believe it is time for our profession to assert the value of the art of medicine.

In a wonderful Christmas Essay published in the *British Medical Journal* in 2008, an American primary care physician, David Loxterkamp, wrote about the doctor–patient relationship, describing how the true lesser spotted empathy can actually breed in this difficult modern environment:

> Most general practitioners I know are reasonably accomplished diagnosticians, skilled technicians, composed professionals and hard workers. We do a job; it pays the bills. Our surgeries are a formidable façade for life's free-for-all: making friends, building businesses, raising families, and growing old together. We have never thought to enforce a degree of separation between the patient and us. In the process, we have learned about human relationships and the larder of trust and gratitude our patients stock on our behalf. Their real value cannot be proved in a laboratory – how can friendship be double blinded or controlled? Yet in this setting, over the space of days or years, patients can discover why they come to see us. We learn how to help. We might even begin to recognise the source of our patients' unhappiness, which lies behind their symptoms and beyond the reach of our diagnostic categories. We offer them recognition, as John Berger taught us in *A Fortunate Man*. We offer something more.
>
> If therapeutic relationships possess a certain unquantifiable magic, it is the magic of hope. When a patient visits the doctor, he or she hopes to be reassured that the lump is not cancer; that the pain will soon end; that a ladder leads from this despair. Hope hinges on the presence of another and the reassurance that yes, we are knowable,

even in the darkest place, yet unknowable to ourselves. Patients and their families need treatment plans to assure them that 'everything is being done' and that the struggle has meaning and purpose in their own terms.

If all this could be accomplished with computerised interviews, health maintenance checklists, and evidence based guidelines, we would not need doctors. Vulnerable patients come to us in desperation. Their fears and insecurities must be met with authority, knowledge, and action. But their humanity requires something more: a handshake, a funny story, our undivided attention – and all that this implies: a doctor who will champion and remain faithful to their cause.

What kind of bird are you? And in this age of organised discontinuity, what kind of bird would you like to be?

References

Loxterkamp D. Why rivers run: on the headwaters of family medicine. *BMJ*. 2008; **337**: a2575.

Watson C. The P value of empathy. *BMJ*. 2005; **330**(7482): 101.

CHAPTER 9

Useful strategies and skills

- Good communicating depends on your attitude.
- Good communication requires skill.
- Skills have a purpose.
- That purpose is to achieve a shared understanding and decision.
- It helps to get the medicine right, too!

Even with the right attitude, sometimes our instinctive skills let us down. To consult well you need to be in the right mood, so the first strategy is to prepare yourself. You must try to generate some enthusiasm and curiosity for the coming encounter. Hopefully, most of what follows is common sense. Imagine yourself in a typical consulting environment. Rearrange the desk a little, have a cup of tea, stretch your legs and take a deep breath. Here goes.

Beginnings

Start by putting your patient at ease. Try to lessen their anxiety and encourage them over their natural diffidence. Some of us are better at this than others, but we can all improve – a smile, a handshake, an individual greeting in the waiting room, perhaps some easy social banter based on previous consultations, a little bit of personal warmth and good eye contact. Try to connect with the human being in front of you.

Your task is to seek out their agenda first, and your own second. When your patient arrives, greet them with appropriate warmth. Try to say as little as possible. Do not say, 'What can I do for you?' and definitely avoid 'What's brought you here?' as you will only get the response of 'The ambulance/the bus/my husband' etc. If you say anything, try 'Well now?' with a quizzical look and an air of expectancy. To begin with, simply encourage your patient – don't interrupt, but do nod, smile, look interested and avoid stopping the flow. This is harder than it sounds, as most of us make a working diagnosis within 20 seconds. With some of our regulars and in most hospital clinics we have made the diagnosis before they come in through the door. When you have made a hypothesis, test it, but be prepared to let go easily and form another hypothesis, and yet another, as necessary. Make an effort to generate several possible hypotheses, and try not to judge too quickly or by appearances. *Thinking, Fast and Slow* (Kahneman, 2011) confirms that we jump to conclusions and then try to confirm our hastily made conclusion. This might work well in some social situations and perhaps when we were hunter-gatherers, but it does not work well in the diagnostic process.

Remind yourself that it is the patient and only the patient who knows the reasons why they have come to see you. If you start on your agenda too soon, you may never discover the fear of cancer, or the fear of the effects of expected therapy, but more importantly you may not discover what it is that the patient actually wants to know. Establishing your patient's agenda early on allows you to negotiate the use of time in the consultation, and to agree on what will be dealt with now and what can be left for another day. It is a much more efficient way of consulting.

It will help you to rehearse the same questions that the patient has asked already.

- Why has this patient come to see you?
- Why now?
- What has happened?
- Why has it happened?
- Why has it happened to him or her?

Put yourself in the patient's shoes as much as you can. This will automatically lead you to real empathy, rather than the much inferior product – sympathy – with which it is so often confused. Avoid using the phrase 'I understand how you must feel' or variations. Although this might seem superficially empathetic, it is patronising and frankly impossible. You will need to listen with genuine interest. This needs to be real and not fake. Work at it. Actively encourage the other person to talk by nodding, smiling and echoing significant words. Show that you are listening and watching (e.g. by saying: 'You look sad today', 'That must have been very frightening' or 'How did that make you feel?'). The educational buzzwords for these behaviours are *'active listening'*.

A good rule is to tell yourself that, at the beginning, the patient is always right – and please remember to let the patient go first. Don't start with a question like 'How's your back?'. Beginnings are very important and will affect the course of the whole meeting, so start open, not closed. Think of the difference between 'Hello, well now?', with a smile and a raised eyebrow, and 'It's your blood pressure, isn't it? Up with the sleeve'. Even the standard opening of 'Hello, what can I do for you?' is controlling, as it implies an action. You may think that this is nit-picking, but do experiment with the effects of various opening gambits. As with chess, you can win or lose the consultation in the first few exchanges.

Starting again

With long-standing patients who you find difficult, it can revolutionise your therapeutic relationship and often your diagnostic acumen if you can clean the slate and start from scratch. You may be surprised by the results. This may be the most important strategy in this whole book.

Take Alice Modell; you have seen her several times in outpatients with essentially medically unexplained symptoms. She was referred under the diagnosis '?Hypothyroid ?MS' and all your investigations have drawn a blank. You are about to send her back to her GP for good when you spot a tear in her eye and decide to try one more time. You say something like, 'Look Mrs Modell, at present we don't know the cause of your symptoms, but perhaps I have missed something, could you tell me what you believe is happening?' She does, you quickly recognise her depressive symptoms, her until now unspoken fear of her brother's motor neurone disease and her apparently genuine descriptions of increasing but intermittent muscle weakness. You don't yet know it but at least now you might: she has early, mild myasthenia gravis.

Ideas, concerns and expectations

Now comes the more difficult bit. You have shaken up your attitude (haven't you?), so now is the time to actively search for your patient's beliefs, ideas, concerns, expectations and feelings, and the effects of these. Try to allow the patient to voice their real concern. This means more than just active listening – it means being interested and wanting to know. To be a good doctor you have to care about people, and if your patients understand that, they will in turn tell you what they care about. Practise picking up on the subtle cues – the sighs, the shoulder shrug, the hasty looking away and the rueful smile.

We must learn to look for the *minimal cues*. Watch your patient carefully and listen to what they say. You must practise true seeing and hearing. Learn to pick up on the cues, both verbal and visual. This is the way into the real agenda, and if you miss the opportunity it may not come again. Watch the patient's facial expression, where they look, and what gestures they make. Do they make eye contact? Watch their posture, muscle tone and breathing. Do they look anxious, sad or angry? Think about their dress and their general appearance. Are they fidgety, relaxed or distant? What might Sherlock Holmes have deduced?

Really listen to them carefully. What does their speech tell you? What are they not saying? How are they saying it? Is their speech too fast, too high-pitched, too slow, or does it have normal rhythm and modulation? Professor Higgins remarked that the moment one Englishman opened his mouth, another Englishman despised him (*Pygmalion*, George Bernard Shaw). We learn a lot the moment our patient says something – their region, their class and ethnic accents being immediately obvious. We obtain further clues about our patient's internal thought patterns by listening to their vocabulary, figures of speech, metaphors and imagery, and their deletions, distortions and generalisations. One of the reasons psychiatrists are often so much more comfortable communicating with patients is that they spend so much of their training practising and developing these skills. They practise observing the minutiae of the consultation including subtle clues to emotions, speech and language, and this is expressly included in the psychiatric 'mental state examination'. While it may not be necessary to record this for every patient, the same principles apply to every patient. But it is an active process which takes effort.

Linguistic experts have studied doctor–patient encounters and identified some common language errors which occur. Here are just a few examples.

- A *deletion* occurs when some detail(s) essential to a complete understanding are missed out by the patient. For example, 'I feel worse.' Worse than what? In what way? Or 'The whole lot are worried about Gramps.' Who in particular? How worried are they? And about what in particular?
- A *distortion* occurs when actual behaviour and events are turned into protective abstract concepts which have no reality of their own. For example, 'I just lost my cool.' What is meant by 'cool'? It does not mean that you can shout and swear at the receptionist. Or 'I'm suffering from my nerves.' What does that mean? That you want more Valium? That you want to see a psychiatrist? Or that the weekly trip to the supermarket is now a nightmare due to increasing agoraphobia?
- A *generalisation* means arguing from the particular to the general in a manner that excludes any possible exceptions to the rule they have made. For example, 'I hate doctors.' Does that mean all doctors, all the time, or just me? Or 'I'm always getting headaches.' Does that mean every week? Every month? Every day? Learn to recognise the patient's internal search and don't interrupt. You need to notice when you have asked the patient a question which they were not expecting, or a chance remark of yours makes them stop and think. Give them time to think, and don't continue with your own agenda until they are ready.

It is very useful to become more adept at demonstrating your grasp of the patient's perspective, as this can really help you to elicit their story. A good strategy is to listen, store up a few social and medical patient cues and then feed them back to show that you are truly interested and hearing what they say. For example, 'I know you sighed early on when I asked if you had any children. Is that important to you?' Or 'I think you are worrying a lot about cancer, but when you say it is in the family, you must not think that all cancers are the same – most of them are not inherited. Is there a cancer that especially worries you?'

You will have to learn to modify your history-taking technique, fashioning it for the individual in front of you. Don't ask too many sequential closed questions, and try to focus on what matters to your patient and to you. Of course you must examine thoroughly but appropriately. This may mean not at all, but don't skimp on necessary examinations because of time pressures. Examinations are a good opportunity to learn things about our patients – and not just that they may have a large liver or an irregular heartbeat. The laying on of hands allows people to talk about deeper fears, and you may find that this phase of the consultation is often the most illuminating of all.

Now think about the beginning again

Learn to speak the patient's language. Do not talk down to them, and avoid using jargon. This implies you have a feel for the patient's language in the first place – you have to work at that. Thinking about preferred styles of communication can help. An example is the Think-Feel-Do model. Patients who are think/doers (like most surgeons and anaesthetists) will prefer a cognitive and practical solution-focused approach. They will respond well to questions like 'What do you think about that?' or 'What shall we do?' On the other hand, people with a predominantly feeling style of social interaction will prefer questions like 'How do you feel about that?' and they will appreciate a more in-depth exploration of their fears and concerns and less emphasis on making a plan. You have to adjust your methodology as you get to know your patient better.

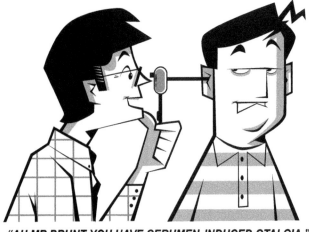

"AH MR BRUNT, YOU HAVE CERUMEN-INDUCED OTALGIA."
"YOU MEAN PAINFUL EARWAX, DOC?"

Patronising 'doctor speak' should be a form of communication that died with the last century, but that may be wishful thinking, as 'complex medical speak' is so much ingrained in doctors that we often don't realise what is jargon to our patients. Keep monitoring your performance and pick out the words and sentences that need translating. You will find that watching recordings of yourself can be particularly illuminating and often chastening. 'Do I really use that much jargon!'

Practise actively encouraging your patient to talk. Nod, smile and echo significant words. Repeat tentatively, in your own words, your understanding of their story. Reflect back in the patient's own words, not only to show that you understand, but also to enable them to hear and understand their own meaning. But be wary of reformulating the patient's words back to them. This can work well, but if you get it wrong the patient may feel alienated and be too afraid to correct you, leading you back to the mismatched agenda. It is important to do this in a highly sensitive and tentative way and seek clarification from the patient. Don't say something too abrupt which paints the patient as demanding or difficult like 'So what you're telling me is you've had panic attacks for years and because they are not getting any better you want to see a psychiatrist?' Try 'So let me see if I've understood you – your panic attacks have been a problem for a long time and now you are wondering whether some specialist advice might help you cope with them better?'

Also, be aware that if you share too much of your thinking with certain patients you are likely to elevate their anxiety, not relieve it. If you mention IBS to some people without yet having a strong conviction this is the case, they may not hear anything else you say as they will fix on this as the diagnosis and be thinking about what it means. A friend of ours went to the doctor with fatigue and vague somatic symptoms. Nothing wrong with her really, just needed reassurance about her life, which was a bit lonely and lacking in direction. However, the doctor did various tests and told her she was wondering about ME. And as there is no test for it, no amount of reassurance will henceforth totally convince her that this is not actually what she has!

Communication tips

You can try making statements which are also good questions. For example, 'I was wondering whether . . .', 'Sometimes I find . . .', 'It occurred to me that . . .', 'My friend John . . .', 'Some people . . .', 'I've known cases where . . .', 'I had a patient once . . .', and so on. Concentrate on asking *open* questions. They are useful for finding out about patients' beliefs, as such questions cannot be answered with a simple yes or no. For example, 'Tell me about . . .', 'What is it like?', 'What are you worried about?', and so on.

The history taking that you have laboriously learned teaches you to ask closed questions, which are useful for obtaining and classifying facts, and for pattern recognition. They are not helpful for eliciting beliefs and feelings, as they tend to increase doctor control and they can only be answered very specifically, often with only a simple yes or no. For example, 'Is it painful?' or 'Are your waterworks all right?' (The last is one of the worst medical euphemisms!)

You are now in the swing of things, so give your patient some encouragement, such as 'Go on' or 'Tell me more', which is the best directive we have ever found – patients always do tell you more. Eye contact and nodding encourage the patient to continue. If you find that your patient will not leave, it may be because you are still fixing them with your gaze and nodding benignly, so they get the message that you wish them to continue talking. Echoing is a good technique for encouraging patients to continue their narrative. This means repeating the last few words of their sentence when they pause, to encourage further revelations; for example, 'Your mother?', 'Afraid?', and so on. You will need to pick up on the cues to do this.

Check what the patient has said. This can be done by giving them your interpretation of their story, thus enabling them to correct any misunderstanding and embellish the story further. This is a good technique, often used by doctors with a military bent. Explain why you are asking a question. This can stimulate unexpected responses.

For example:

> Dr: 'The reason I asked about wind and bloating was that I was wondering about irritable bowel syndrome.'
> Patient: 'Oh, my sister's got that, and she said that's what I've got, but my mother reckons it's an ulcer.'

Or, of course, there is the studied use of silence. This is often frightening to young doctors who, every time there is a pause, feel uncomfortable and duty-bound to say something, however inane. Try allowing pauses. The patient will invariably fill them if you wait long enough. Silence is something all doctors should cultivate. Not only does it actually mean we get more information but patients perceive doctors who allow pauses for them to talk as being more understanding. Interactions with patients where the doctor actually says (and does) very little often rate as some of the most satisfying for patients. The ability to talk about their problems and concerns is frequently our patient's main reason for seeing you in whatever setting of medicine, though they often do not realise this themselves.

That is a lot to digest. Another truth may have dawned on you. You will need to practise, watch yourself, get some feedback and practise again. Good medical communication takes a lot of practice, but like doing anything skilful well, it is worth it in the long run, and the long run is your medical career.

The second half of the encounter

At this stage we should perhaps remind you that this is a book for doctors. Good communication skills and bad medicine are sadly increasingly common bedfellows – don't forget the science that you have been taught. This book is about communicating that hard-learned science effectively, so by this stage of the consultation we hope you have got the medical content right. If so, now you must learn how to negotiate with the patient.

The doctor should go first. You have to outline your position and your reasons. Try thinking aloud, and state your position. Be honest. Give the patient a few choices. Ask them what they think. Reinforce their good ideas and counter the bad ones, but be careful what you say. For example, 'Don't worry' means that worrying is an option, 'Won't' means might, 'Can't' means could and 'Shouldn't' means probably will. Use questions as statements. For example, 'Do you ever think you'll come off the tranquillisers?'

Again remember to watch the patient's internal search. If you do not see the patient looking as if they accept what you say, continue to negotiate. Watch for 'non-verbal leakage'. This may sound like a pool of muddy water forming round your patient, but it is actually the discrepancy between what your patient says and what their non-verbal behaviour is indicating. For example, 'No, I'm not depressed', while sitting with shoulders slumped, a sad fixed expression and exuding gloom. Or 'Yes, I will probably try the tablets', while breaking eye contact and squirming in the chair. You have to act on these cues in order to be effective. For example, 'I know you say you are not depressed, but you do look it to me. Are you sure there isn't something I can help with?'

You must try to involve your patients in the decision making. This may mean countering their fallacious arguments and erroneous beliefs, and reinforcing those beliefs that are helpful to the outcome. Try to foster patient autonomy and increase patient self-reliance. Remember that you are more powerful than you think you are, so use your power carefully (*see* Chapter 2). For example, should you sit behind the desk instead of to one side of it? Should you fill your consulting area with potentially frightening medical paraphernalia? Don't let your personal attitudes intrude too much, even though you are now aware that they are ultimately guiding your actions. You must be prepared on occasion to admit to uncertainty, and this may not be easy for either you or your patient. Uncertainty is all-pervading – it is the worm in the apple of perfection. Your inner self is always in doubt, but this is the truth about being a doctor. Develop your humanity and learn to realise that uncertainty comes with the territory. Dealing with uncertainty is one of the hardest skills to learn in medicine; the earlier the phase of the illness the greater the uncertainty. An experienced GP will cope with uncertainty much better than a newly qualified F1.

You can also use shepherding techniques. For example, if you do not want the patient to go to an osteopath, you can call him 'a bloke that tweaks backs for £50 a time'. Or if you do wish the patient to go, the osteopath becomes 'a colleague with more training in manipulation than me'. Another steering method is to use presuppositions, such as 'Do you think you will find it easier to stop smoking all at once or to gradually cut down over a fortnight?' Or you can use the 'My friend John technique'; for example, 'I remember someone else who did what you are thinking of and found out the hard way . . .'

Learn to use appropriate delivery, which is how you say something, not what you say. Start by breaking information down into manageable chunks. Keep pausing and checking. Is the patient following what you are saying? Pace (the speed of delivery) is important. Try to match the patient's rate of speech. Eye contact is important.

Keep watching for those minimal cues. Try to match the patient's language of self-expression. For example, 'You said you were "absolutely knackered". Don't worry, an operation like you have just had makes you feel that way.'

Think about reframing statements/questions to alter the perspective. For example, a 3-year-old boy seen in paediatric triage because he is 'wilfully' scratching his baby sister's face could easily be labelled 'attention-seeking', which could make things worse. What if he were labelled 'attention-needing'? Framing is a commonly used technique for selling treatments.

Remember that understanding of the words 'common', 'possible' and 'rare' can vary, and the use of percentages or other figures may be interpreted in very different ways. For example, patients are more likely to take a treatment such as simvastatin if they are told that it will reduce their risk of having another heart attack by a third than if they are told that it will reduce their actual risk from 12% to 8%. They will be even less accepting if they are told that the number of patients who would need to be treated for 10 years in order to prevent one attack is 25. The important task is to convey such information in ways that are meaningful to the individual patient while not manipulating the message too disingenuously. This is an area of intense research, and the reading list at the end of the book might be helpful. There is a rash of decision-making aids appearing, and their quality varies enormously.

At this juncture, a word of caution should be given about a ghastly new verb that has crept into the medical vocabulary, namely consent. As in: 'Go and consent Mrs Arthur for the ^{131}I treatment.' This is a doctor-centred behaviour and bears no relationship to the true spirit of informed consent. Informed consent is a two-way process, based on a shared understanding, checked by you, and a true involvement in management with genuine option sharing. Imagine the woman in agonising labour asked to consent to an urgent C-section. Exactly how much informed consent is she capable of at this point? The signature is not worth the paper it is written on.

Take a breather at this stage of the chapter.

Now think about practising the second half of the consultation. It is our experience that enlightenment does not come all at once to most of us. Getting the first half of the consultation right will give you the springboard to perform the second half well, but the tasks and skills involved are very different. If you are a golfer it is the difference between driving and round-the-green play – all part of the same game, but very different actions are required.

Just as an exercise, let us change tack for a while and think about those really difficult areas that involve trying to change our patients' entrenched and unhealthy behaviours. Medical Royal Colleges and Government want doctors to help patients give up the fags, lose the flab, get fitter, or even just take the tablets that they should be taking. The Government is clear that this is our responsibility. We think they are wrong, but how can we at least put our patients on the right track? Here are four linked strategies to think about.

- *Make things easy*. People are more likely to do things if there are fewer things to do, if they fit in with their existing lifestyle and if they have the necessary resources.
- *Think of the context*. People are more likely to do things if they do them with other people, if they are reminded at the time to do them, if they know someone might be likely to check to see whether they have done them, and if the people with whom they live and work are willing to help them.
- *Think of the patient's perceptions*. People are more likely to do things that seem important, and when they understand why they should do them and how to do them. If they really believe in your advice, they will follow it, and they are more likely to do things if their anxiety level is raised moderately but not too high.
- *Think of the relationship*. People are more likely to do things if they have helped to decide that it would be beneficial, if they have promised to do these things and if they have faith in you as their doctor, especially if they think that you like and respect them, and if they are rewarded for doing these things.

Now let us go back to the second half of the consultation and think about the crucial explanation phase. Remember that this book is about learning to share in the consultation, *and the goal is to reach a shared understanding and a shared decision* with your patient. This is a significant step further than a simple explanation.

First you *must* elicit the patient's beliefs. You cannot share unless you have something to share. This sounds breathtakingly obvious, but many doctors who are observed in video recordings for assessment purposes are not actually doing it. You have to recognise that the whole consultation, particularly the process of eliciting, organising and reflecting the information that the patient gives you, is an experience from which the patient can learn – as can you. You can practise translating and sharing your medical knowledge honestly and with respect for the patient. This means maintaining or enhancing your patient's autonomy by respecting and not patronising him or her.

Here we move to a higher level of skilfulness. Try to clarify how much information your patient actually wants. Encouraging the patient to ask you at least one or two questions is a good start. This needs practice. It is a good idea not to reassure the patient too soon, as this can be interpreted as rejection or a lack of knowledge. Bear in mind that while an explanation is a one-way process, the goal is a shared understanding, which is a two-way behaviour.

Practise presenting information without using jargon, and instead use short words and sentences as specifically as possible. Remember that the order in which information is given is important. Patients recall best what they are told first. Repeat important pieces of information. Now a caveat about avoiding jargon – this can make you sound very patronising, which is the reason it is a skill and must be carefully judged. Trainees sometimes get this wrong in their practical exams and in trying to avoid sounding overly paternalistic end up sounding belittling and undermining. Don't forget that patients are just people who want information in a way they can understand.

A good technique to learn and practise is 'explicit categorisation'. For example, 'I am going to tell you what I think is wrong, what I expect to happen, and which treatment I suggest.' Again this may seem a bit military, but it is very effective. Get into the habit of using leaflets, tapes, DVDs, websites, etc. Read or listen to them first, as you may find that you disagree with them vehemently! Ideally, write them yourself.

Actively encourage feedback, check your attitude again, and regularly check your patient's understanding, not least because it will probably increase your own. It is bad practice to give too much information, and don't get carried away by your own verbosity. A patient staring out of the window at the squirrels is a sure sign that you have gone on too long. Remember that much of what we tell patients they forget immediately, even if they understood or were listening in the first place. They tend to remember what matters to them; this is often not what matters to you.

When negotiating about treatment, specific questions are helpful. For example, 'How have you been using your medication?', 'Tell me when you take it' and 'What do you find the problems with the treatment are?' A word of warning, though. 'Why' questions tend to put patients on the defensive, and there is a tendency to invent answers.

You will find that it will help to (metaphorically) climb a few steps down from your pedestal – in other words, try not to be too distanced from your patient because of your need to be professional. Remember to use similar phrases to the patient, and some of their own descriptions, and you will find it instructive (and sometimes cathartic) to share a little of yourself from time to time. For example, 'I had a heart operation and it shook me up' or 'Migraines are bloody awful, aren't they?'

It will help the whole process if you can demonstrate some understanding and empathy. Empathy, as we have already touched on, is a much abused concept. The idea is to identify mentally with the patient and so fully comprehend them. This is fine so long as you realise it is only an aim that can help you to communicate with your patient. It may be impossible to empathise fully with someone, and you will find some groups especially difficult. For example, how can middle-class doctors really empathise with drug-abusing teenagers? We can be compassionate and we can care for them, but the vast majority of us will be unable to truly empathise with them. The medical communication skill we call empathy is about *trying to understand*. We might not succeed but we should make a concerted effort to try to imagine their situation in order to communicate effectively with them. The 'common nice mumble' is essentially effortless pleasantry unlike the much rarer bird, the 'lesser spotted empathy'. You are trying to be that bird.

Achieving a shared understanding does not mean always getting the patient to agree with you. It means that in order to achieve a genuine sharing you may have to agree with them. This may make you uneasy, and on occasions you may have to soften your views in order to try to keep a dialogue going. You cannot share with a monologue.

Now let us recap some of the essentials.

- Determine the reasons for the patient's attendance at the outset. This then allows you both to set the agenda; that is, what you will cover today and what can be reasonably left for another occasion. This is a genuinely time-conserving strategy.
- Determine the patient's own ideas, concerns and expectations before you attempt an explanation. In this way you will reduce

the risk of a 'dysfunctional' consultation, and the explanation will become tailored to that individual patient.
• Use each consultation as part of a learning circle. Some tasks can be achieved over a series of consultations. The adoption of these methods may also change patients' expectations about the appropriate use of time and resources.

Remember that there are other things to do as well. In all of this communicating you will need to record information (both clinical and patient-centred) effectively. This is another skill that needs much practice and is not easy. Structured dictation helps, and when the speech translation software improves this will be even more useful.

To be an effective physician, you will need to obtain as much information as possible about the availability of resources in your field. Try not to prescribe prematurely, expensively or inappropriately. For juniors we think this is even more difficult. As doctors become more confident in their abilities and more experienced they may be more able to see the bigger picture and adopt a watch and wait approach. Trainees should be encouraged to think carefully about exactly what they are hoping to accomplish by prescribing.

Another task is to help the patient to appreciate the costs and benefits of concordance and non-concordance. It will benefit both you and the patient to keep the treatment as simple as possible, and remember to share management strategies and decisions. The human capacity for self-repair should also encourage you to bear in mind the adage 'Do as much nothing as possible'.

To use time effectively, all of these skills need to be practised and honed. Self-observation is essential, and peer observation is very helpful.

General communication skills

Here are a few tips and thoughts about general communication skills. Some studies have shown that a female style of communication results in more sharing, others that men use time more efficiently. The good news for both sexes is that they are both as likely to be able to demonstrate a patient-centred approach in observed recordings. This suggests that patient-centred medicine is not a natural communication gift, and it must be learned by both sexes.

You can learn the skills of appropriate control, including the judicious use of doctor authority to control speech flow, and the appropriate use of negative non-verbal behaviour (*not* looking at the patient will tend to staunch the flow). Closing the patient's notes, or turning the computer screen away, can signal the end of the consultation. Wearing a dinner-jacket tends to speed patients up a bit, but cannot be used too often. Standing up and holding the door open will stop all but the most dedicatedly self-obsessed. Removing the chair is a last resort. Feigning a fit is a desperation measure.

At the strategic level you, the doctor, should strive to create an environment that facilitates the exchange of information; for example, seating position, not having a big chair for the doctor and a small chair for the patient, ambience, accessibility, dress, décor, and so on. As we have said, be friendly and attentive, and adopt an informal style. However, be wary of the overuse of first names – it is easy to be patronising. The 'I am Lulu, fly me' style that is now universal in NHS wards is not always appropriate for complex doctor–patient interactions. After a while it is not unreasonable to ask your patient if they mind being called by their first name. Many patients quite like being addressed in this way but will never call you by yours. However, beware the patient's notes in this context, as using the first name indicated is fraught with dangers. For example, Mr Cyril Blodwin may hate being called Cyril, and when with friends will only answer to Jack, so by not checking you may have been blithely annoying him for a decade.

It helps to use plural pronouns to indicate partnership. For example, 'I hope you agree. Shall we meet again in two weeks to see how you are getting on?' Use self-disclosure to establish trust and common ground. For example, 'Yes, I know you must be frightened. I am terrified of the dentist.' Make comments that are provisional rather than dogmatic. For example, 'I think your blood pressure probably needs treatment. Here is a leaflet to read. I would like you to come back to discuss the treatment and what you think about it' is preferable to 'Your blood pressure is up. Take these tablets – the nurse will explain.'

Try to respond descriptively, not judgementally. For example, on being asked the question 'What about my knees, doctor?', the response 'I think you have some wear and tear, possibly a little early arthritis' is OK, but 'You're too fat and that's why you have knee pain' is a bit bald – dress up the message. Make comments that are related to the problem(s) rather than to controlling the patient. For example:

> I think, since your heart attack, your heart is under a little strain. You will feel better with some fluid tablets, but you will need some time off work because you will need some time for the heart to recover. I will make you an appointment for some rehabilitation which will help you and get you back to work quicker. Here is a leaflet about what I mean.

This is better than:

> You must stay off work until I tell you. Go for rehabilitation treatment, this will be good for you, and here are some water tablets to take every morning.

Learn to recognise the effect of your own behaviour on your patient. Are you frightening? Do you inspire trust? Do your patients come back to you? What do they tell you about yourself? Learn to recognise, interpret and use your feelings. If you are feeling uneasy and anxious, is your patient feeling that way, too? If you are getting angry, are they, too? Learn to recognise and deal with your own stress. You could read Samuel Shem's *The House of God* (1978). Talk to your friends and to yourself (but not too much of the latter!).

With regard to waiting times, most patients don't mind waiting if they are warned that you will be late. Always acknowledge your lateness and make some gesture of apology – hardly anyone will then still object.

According to the Medical Protection Society most complaints are due to a failure of effective communication and one of the biggest is the failure of doctors to realise how important it is to be up front when there is a mistake and say sorry. Covering up mistakes or trying to ignore them makes patients angrier than acknowledging them and apologising. Patients also want reassurance the same mistake will not be made again.

Strategies and skills that are helpful when using desktop computers and note-taking

Strategically positioned computer screens should be visible to the patient and a focus for sharing information. A study of MRCGP candidates in 2000 demonstrated that this actually occurs in less than 10% of surgeries. Note-writing and data entry should be kept to a minimum while the patient is present, because they can hinder communication. A useful rule is to read the notes before the consultation and to write them up afterwards. The increasing use of electronic records does allow easier use of the record while one is actually consulting, the quality of the data being the most important factor.

The computer is only a tool – don't let it dictate the agenda (although it does). Read coding (and soon the next type of codes), now essential to modern medical data recording, constrains and limits the boundaries of the consultation. It also tends to emphasise the biomedical model of disease at the expense of the more realistic social and emotional basis of most medical encounters. Computers and their software pose a great threat to the 'art' of medicine, and we as a profession need to devise ways of redressing the balance very soon.

It is sad but true that many patients will take advice from the computer screen more avidly than they will take it from you. Learn to share understanding and clarify the story by using and discussing the information on the screen together. Never write in the notes or enter into the computer record anything you would not wish your patient to see. Remember that patients have the right of access to their notes and any data about them that are held on computer. All computer systems have the facility to record sensitive information (e.g. previous termination) in such a way as not to be displayed for general view (e.g. to the dismay of the new boyfriend).

Children and their parents

You will quickly learn that children from as young as three are capable of quite complex thought and communication. Many children are more on the ball than their parents. In the clinic they will usually defer to their parents, but this does not mean that they are not listening and understanding. Always take the child into account when giving any explanation, and watch their reaction as well as that of the parent.

It is essential to realise that parents are programmed to worry about their children. They usually fear the worst and are suspicious of doctors underestimating the severity of the illness. Doctors can easily misinterpret this as over-concern or neurosis. For example, consider the scenario of a young mother with a 6-month-old baby with some mild vomiting and diarrhoea, already settling by the time she sees you. You believe, with considerable justification, that this is a common, non-worrying and self-limiting condition. However, the mother believes that her baby could be very ill, and specifically that her vomiting could induce a ruptured blood vessel in the stomach and that she could bleed to death – a belief she has acquired from watching a recent soap on television. After the initial exchange and examination, which reveal that the baby is neither ill nor dehydrated, she has only vomited twice and the stools are loose but not watery, the exchange goes something like this:

Mother: I am very worried about her vomiting.

Doctor: Don't worry, she isn't dehydrated. Her nappies are still wet, aren't they?

Mother: Yes, but . . .

Doctor: Well, I wouldn't worry – give me a ring if she is not settling or her nappies dry out, OK?

Mother: But the vomiting, doctor?

Doctor: She is OK, honestly.

Mother: But are you sure? She is so little.

Doctor: Yes, of course I am sure. Don't worry; I've seen lots of babies.

Mother [increasingly distressed]: But could she die, doctor?

Doctor [increasingly frustrated]: She is not dehydrated; she will be fine. You must not get yourself so worked up.

Mother [in tears]: I suppose you are right, doctor.

She leaves hurriedly. You are bewildered and think she is anxious and difficult. You make some remark to your colleague about young Mrs M being in a right state about a perfectly healthy baby, and blame it on the lack of family support. This is a truly dysfunctional consultation. How might you have prevented it?

You could have avoided this situation by seeking out her concerns. We must always seek out parents' concerns. They may be bizarre, and as we usually couldn't guess them we must ask. In this example you could have said, 'You look really worried. What is it you are frightened of?' The mother might then have told you.

Parents need help to understand their children's illnesses and to get the right perspective. This means that we have to explain clearly, and to give and share information which is consistent with the parents' concerns, beliefs and expressed needs. Special skills are needed for gaining the confidence of children, and these vary with age, gender and temperament. Try to learn from colleagues who have such skills, as there is an art to winning a child's confidence and then persuading them to talk openly to you. As a rough rule of thumb, children respond surprisingly well to being treated in an adult manner, and after the initial surprise they enjoy being involved in the conversation.

The two- or three-way consultations impose a greater strain on our communication skills (e.g. the weeping mum whose two toddlers are spraying ethyl chloride on the new baby's nose and rummaging about in a sharps box which should have been removed weeks ago, while simultaneously screaming that they must go to the loo now). We have no easy solutions for this all too familiar scenario, and welcome suggestions. What we have learned is to try to put everything out of reach of children, but somehow this never works. We have tried staring doe-eyed into the collapsing patient's eyes, forcibly exuding warm sprays of empathy, while inwardly screaming for an electrified crèche several miles away. Sometimes the temptation to chastise the little darlings verbally or physically is almost overwhelming, but it doesn't help the mother. Calm support for her, if possible bolstering her own parental authority, is really the order of the day. Reception staff with black belts in judo can sometimes be cajoled into looking after the children for long enough for the mother to get the prescription for Prozac, but the only way to help her properly is either to try to find another time when the kids can be left somewhere else, or to visit her at home and risk that rising-damp feeling as you sink into the sofa just vacated by the nappy-less Tarquin.

Consulting with family members present

Good and bad communication strategies with more than one person present

Good:

- keeping confidentiality issues high on your agenda
- greeting each individual including children in such a way as to encourage their participation
- being on the lookout for and acknowledging the emotions expressed (positive and negative)
- trying to control monopolisation and limiting persistent interruptions
- emphasising the positive.

Not so good:

- stopping the story too soon
- letting one individual regularly speak for another
- taking sides
- offering advice without fully exploring the problem
- leaving the computer screen notes of one partner available for another to view.

The dynamics of communication are very different when a third party or more parties participate, but the central aim remains to achieve a shared understanding based on your and their medical knowledge; it is just harder.

The central issue can be dissected by thinking of agendas; but whose? There is that of the 'patient' (and it may not always be entirely clear who that is), the family member's and the doctor's. Take the mother and 14-year-old sexually eager daughter scenario, which is a very common one. The fact that mother is there usually indicates that her agenda is probably closely linked to her daughter's and that there is unlikely to be a conflict. Both want the pill, for it to be done properly, and both want a bit of professional input to legitimise the socially normal but technically illegal decision. Then what about the Gillick competent consultation? Here an angry mum comes with a sheepish daughter brandishing a packet of the pill that you have prescribed; who is the patient here? And whose agenda is paramount? This is a difficult interaction as you are aware. Your own agenda becomes very important here, which will be influenced by your beliefs – religious, ethical and practical ones. The consultation will be guided by who you deem to be the patient. Most will choose the daughter, but for some it will be the mother, and thus her agenda that holds centre stage.

So how can we oil the wheels, as it were, in such a situation? There is likely to be a lot of tension in the room, so diffusing this probably unhelpful atmosphere must be a priority. Listening professionally is usually the best way to do it, as this will allow you to establish their agendas and so guide your subsequent interventions. It is a good strategy in all three-way consultations to let the most eager participant begin; in this case it will probably be wise to let Mother have her say first. Listen, don't judge, and watch the daughter's non-verbal behaviour to get a clue as to the level and type of emotion that is uppermost. When you have truly allowed her to express her expectations, her concerns and gauged the depth of feeling, it is time to let the daughter have her say. You must treat her as an equal and at all costs respect her vulnerability and her confidentiality. Don't, for example, have the computer screen of her recent medical history visible for her mother to scrutinise. Consider whether speaking to her by herself for a few minutes might be helpful. She is young, and this meeting may set her expectations of the medical profession for the rest of her life, so there is a lot at stake. It is only after you have understood the differing viewpoints that you can have a role in the resolution, and of course the very act of being a sort of calming referee is of itself often very therapeutic and may be all that is needed.

The takeaway message is that in all interactions with family members it is the various agendas that matter.

Cross-cultural issues

These skills are difficult to acquire and are really beyond the scope of this book, but many regions are experiencing a large increase in the number of such consultations. We must confess to a lack of specific expertise in this area, but a few strategies come to mind. The first relates to the use of translators. A third party will lengthen the consultation, so you will need more time (often much easier said than done), but more subtly you must be aware that your patient may omit important parts of the history because of embarrassment or worries about confidentiality. If the translator is related to the patient, family dynamics come into play. With all of these variables it can be rather like consulting while wearing a motorcycle helmet with a dirty visor. Familiar signals may not mean the same thing, eye contact may be abhorred, a nod may not indicate acceptance, and so on, so your only resort is to keep checking your patient's understanding as best you can. There are now several good texts on this subject, and you should read at least one of them.

Use of the telephone

The telephone is now ubiquitous. In some surgeries more consultations are conducted by telephone than face to face. This form of communication is more difficult, and there are fewer cues, but all the basic rules apply. As the assessment is based solely on the history, and the management plan cannot be reinforced with non-verbal cues, it is especially important to be systematic in covering all of the issues.

In the most authoritative recent review article on telephone consulting (McKinstry *et al.*, 2009), the authors suggest that the telephone should be primarily used for follow-up appointments, and for the management of long-term conditions when diagnostic assessment has already been undertaken. The newish (2014) 111 telephone advice service is now with us. All types of acute medical problems are now triaged and managed via the phone and unsurprisingly there have been many problems and some evidence of an increase in referrals to the emergency department. This may be inevitable in a system with few doctors.

It has been suggested that training in telephone consultation skills should focus on the following:
- active listening and structured medical history taking
- frequent clarification and paraphrasing (to ensure that the messages have been conveyed in both directions)
- picking up cues (e.g. pace, pauses, change in voice intonation)
- providing opportunities to ask questions
- offering patient education
- sharing understanding
- sharing decisions
- arranging appropriate review
- documentation.

When does communication go wrong?

1 When we are rushed.
2 When we are interrupted.
3 When we get the wrong notes or computer-screen display to start with.
4 When more than one patient consults at once (e.g. mother and children, or husband and wife).
5 When the patient is angry (and when we are angry).
6 When we have a difficult patient.
7 When the patient was expecting to see a different doctor.
8 During evening surgeries! One study found that consultations in the evening are three times more likely to go wrong than those in morning surgeries.
9 When the relationship is difficult.
10 When there are real communication problems (e.g. language, speech, idiom, etc.).
11 *Most important of all*, when we don't find out why our patient has really come to see us and what it is that matters to them.

References

Kahneman D. *Thinking, Fast and Slow*. New York: Farrar, Straus and Giroux; 2011.

McKinstry B, Watson P, Pinnock H, *et al.* Telephone consulting in primary care: a triangulated qualitative study of patients and providers. *Br J Gen Pract.* 2009; **59**: 209–18.

Shem S. *The House of God*. New York: Dell Publishing; 1978.

CHAPTER 10

Wider communication and ethical issues

'Whole patient medicine'

At its most basic, the concept of 'whole patient medicine' requires doctors to think of other illness, such as a sore throat in a diabetic patient, or a patient presenting with a red eye but who is also severely crippled by arthritis. These descriptions are already clearly reductionist – a characteristic of Western medicine. The more embracing or holistic concepts of the ill person are more usually associated with Eastern thought, or in current Western society with the practitioners of fringe medicine. That this is an ethical issue relates to the effect on the individual. Reductionism and disease orientation encourage the development of teaching such as 'Go and see the liver failure in bed seven and tell me what clinical signs you detect.'

There is an inherent conflict between the disease-based medical model and the more socio/psychological models that emphasise unwellness or maladaptation of a person in the context of their family and society. The reductionist model may be at its least helpful when it comes to mental health. Increasingly, there is a shift away from the determination to categorise everyone neatly within an ICD-10 code to a more dimensional approach looking at symptoms and degree of impairment. Perhaps the same might be applicable to other areas of medicine where the truth is that most diagnoses are much less certain than we like to think.

Avoiding the worst excesses of this conflict requires doctors to make an effort to see their patients as individuals and to consider the whole person and their medical problems in an embracing rather than exclusive style. This is more difficult for the specialist, and it is an ethical reason for regretting the demise of the generalist in hospitals.

Shared decision making and informed consent

The current enthusiasm for shared decision making is a logical development of the earlier concept of informed consent, itself a relatively new and transatlantic concept, having been first mentioned in a Californian supreme court in 1957. There is no doubt that in our present society the idea of informed consent remains very important, very necessary and relates fundamentally to the ability of the medical profession to communicate well with patients. A brief consideration of the history of communication in medicine will indicate what new ideas these are.

The most influential figure in shaping the relationship between doctor and patient over the last 3000 years has probably been Hippocrates. His famous but rather weird oath makes no reference at all to a doctor's duty to converse with patients. In fact, in *Decorum* he admonishes doctors to 'perform their duties calmly and adroitly, concealing most things from the patient . . . revealing nothing of the patient's future or present condition'. Plato, in several of his writings, stated quite categorically that doctors had a right to employ lies for good and noble purposes. This Greek ethic was entrenched in the best of motives – it was thought to be necessary, as the belief was that without respect for medical authority there could be no cure. The idea of the patient participating in decision making was seen as counterproductive. The doctor knew what was best for the patient. The main tenets of Greco-Roman medicine were that patients must honour doctors, for the latter received their authority from God, and that patients must have faith in their doctors and must promise obedience. After being around for so long, such ideas do not disappear quickly. How many doctors do you know who still hold views like this?

In the eighteenth and nineteenth centuries a few isolated luminaries suggested educating and involving patients. John Gregory, Professor of Medicine at Edinburgh, was a notable example, and Benjamin Rush, a famous American contemporary of Gregory, held similar views but, like Gregory, favoured deception whenever enlightenment was not equal to the task. They were both essentially pragmatists, seeking the most effective doctor–patient relationship for therapeutic ends, and not so very concerned about educating patients to share the burdens of decision making.

Some patients were beginning to get a little restless by the middle of the nineteenth century. John Stuart Mill, the famous libertarian, put it quite succinctly in 1859: 'Over himself, his own body and mind, the individual is sovereign.' It took another 100 years for this idea to permeate through to a significant number of the medical profession.

As well as believing that telling patients too much is bad for them, many doctors also continue to believe that patients will not want to know or to participate in the process of decision making. See Fowler *et al.* (2013) for their article 'How patient centered are medical decisions?' Turns out, still not very.

Clinicians can improve participation by modest changes in how they communicate with patients. Doctors sometimes believe they are considering their patients' values and preferences in the treatment options they offer, but this often involves incorrect assumptions (Mulley *et al.*, 2012).

Until very recently this assumption was particularly rife in mental health. There was a prevailing attitude that people in hospital, especially those detained under the Mental Health Act, would be unable and unwilling to engage in any discussion about their treatment or future pathway. Of course it now seems obvious to most that this is nonsense. Even people who are profoundly mentally unwell have ideas, concerns and expectations about their treatment and need their doctors to give them an appropriate amount of information in a form they can access and understand. Many will have a clear wish to participate in shared decision making and in many instances this will lead to a better therapeutic partnership and outcomes.

A great deal of emphasis is put on training psychiatrists to be good at this shared approach now. But aside from primary care there seems to be very little time or energy devoted to it in other training schemes. If patients with treatment-resistant schizophrenia who have been institutionalised for 20 years can actively and successfully participate in a true dialogue about their care, why should we assume that other patients cannot or will not?

On the other hand, the issue of coercion is particularly acute in these patients. Some might argue that patients in this situation cannot give truly informed consent as the power differential is too great. Any potential for them to move forward is determined by the extent to which they engage with their team. Doctors need to be fully aware of this and do all they can to ensure patients can meaningfully participate in their care, including, where appropriate, directing changes to their treatment or declining it altogether. The issue of capacity is obviously important here.

Today the informed consent industry is a growth area, but the product is often rather shoddy. Many doctors still think that telling patients too much is bad for them, despite the existence of overwhelming evidence to the contrary. In fact patients actually become less anxious if they are adequately informed about major surgical procedures, nasty invasive tests, unpleasant treatments and dangerous drugs.

The American researchers Greenfield and colleagues (1985) turned this conundrum on its head. They asked themselves the question: If doctors do not inform patients too well, what will happen if we teach patients to ask searching questions of their doctors and to negotiate decisions relating to their own care? They took three groups of patients from a Californian hospital – people with peptic ulcers, people with high blood pressure and people with diabetes – and using a randomised technique, they split each group into two, and trained one group to ask appropriate questions and negotiate decisions. They then measured outcomes. So what happened? Lo and behold, in the experimental groups the blood sugar level improved significantly, the blood pressure dropped significantly, ulcers improved more quickly and the patients were happier and liked the involvement. If these results had been achieved by a new diabetic agent the pharmaceutical companies would have been ecstatic, but all that was in fact needed was some additional two-way communication.

In 1994, when this book was first published, the anaesthetic department at the Freeman Hospital in Newcastle-upon-Tyne set up a project on postoperative pain relief and the use of self-administering injection pumps. In summary, the patients were using the pumps but were provided with little information and experienced only limited pain relief, although marginally better than that obtained with conventional drug administration. Those patients who received information and explanations from the staff were then given total control of the injection pump containing opiate, etc., and reported dramatic and almost total relief of pain. Again, a dose of communication gave patients control over their own suffering, with gratifying results.

The fact that informed consent and shared decision making are now such major issues is good for patients, as they are offered more information than ever before. Surgeries overflow with leaflets on every conceivable subject, hospital outpatient departments have printed sheets on most known diseases and procedures, bookshops have huge sections on health and illness, and magazines, radio phone-ins, television programmes and telephone helplines all devote an ever increasing amount of coverage to health-related matters. CD-ROMs, DVDs and the Internet are now here to stay.

While rewriting this chapter in 2008 Peter used an Internet search engine to look for references on communication in medicine – there were over 100,000 entries. Now in early 2014, in a search lasting 0.27 of a second there are 27 million. As early as 1996, a patient of Peter's with chronic pancreatitis came with a sheaf of printouts from Medline, and asked to be referred to Dundee, as he had just read their paper on stenting the duct. This was extremely unusual behaviour then; it is commonplace now. Whether doctors like it or not, there is a change in society's attitude. Although individually patients still tend to adopt a passive role, society as a whole expects the medical profession to educate, inform and involve. The well-known journalist John Illman (2000) has produced a booklet for the Association of the British Pharmaceutical Industry (ABPI) entitled *The Expert Patient*, in which he lists a nine-point patient's code. A slightly shortened version is given here.

1   Prepare for the consultation. Write down your symptoms and worries and take the list with you.
2   Be honest, but don't leave things to chance in the hope that they will suddenly disappear. Delay can be dangerous.
3   Be polite. Doctors are not Superman and Superwoman, but ordinary people trying to do a good job. Just like everyone else, they feel more inclined to make an effort for people who show appreciation.
4   Respect your doctor. No one likes to be told how to do their job. An increasing number of patients are demanding treatment from doctors on the basis of information from the Internet or the mass media. By all means discuss any information you have gathered, but ask your doctor which treatment he or she would want in your circumstances.
5   Listen carefully. Take written notes or, even better – if your doctor does not mind – record the consultation.

6   Don't be afraid to ask questions. You may help your doctor to improve his or her communication skills by asking questions if you don't understand the information.

7   Ask about groups that know about your condition. Ask your doctor for details of relevant support groups.

8   Don't be afraid to ask for a second opinion, but be polite about it.

9   Don't be afraid to complain. Again, this is your right, but be polite. Most complaints against doctors are about rudeness and poor communication.

The right to be heard implies the *time* to be heard. This is a stark fact – many patients find the constraints of short appointments and rushed outpatient appointments irksome and frustrating. There is evidence that patients make very accurate assessments of how much time they will need with doctors in a primary care setting, as of course they are aware of their own agenda. When patients have been allowed to choose short, medium or long appointments, on the whole this has increased satisfaction for both parties. In ideal, well-financed medical systems, time is not a problem. It is a further reason why many patients attend fringe medical practitioners – they have bought the time.

Most patients in the UK and America are unused to overt rationing, but in the UK covert rationing is the norm, as the demise of the NHS and the rise in managed care have imposed the harsh reality on all. Consumerism, choice, autonomy and rationing produce dissatisfaction and conflict with the medical profession.

True consent is increasingly regarded as a right, and if this right is seen to be denied or infringed, litigation ensues more and more frequently. UK law is still somewhat unclear, but the Sidaway case in England and the Moyes case in Scotland are the most commonly cited precedents. The law does not yet seem to require that fully informed consent should be obtained in all cases, but it does require that important material risks should be disclosed and that all of the patient's questions are answered truthfully. As a criterion for what constitutes a material risk, the 'Bolam' principle applies. Put simply, this states that a doctor should act 'in accordance with a practice accepted as proper by a body of responsible and skilled medical opinion' (Lord Diplock). Lord Templeman has emphasised that the amount of medical information that is offered to patients cannot be consistent:

A patient may make an unbalanced judgement because he is deprived of information. A patient may also make an unbalanced judgement if he is provided with too much information and is made aware of possibilities which he is not capable of assessing because of his lack of medical training, his prejudices, or his personality.

The impact of the new European legislation on human rights has yet to be tested.

There has been a seismic shift in attitude and opinion since the 'Bristol case', in which two cardiac surgeons were vilified and humiliated. Although this was partly on account of their poor surgical performance in certain difficult operations on small children, the major complaint by parents concerned the lack of openness and honesty about the chances of success. The expectations of the public with regard to truthful communication by doctors about treatment risks and benefits have never been higher. The discomforting fact for doctors is that much of the information on success rates which was kept from the Bristol parents still remains hidden in many units up and down the UK.

These awful experiences highlight the fact that achieving true informed consent is fraught with difficulties. Most consent is a long way from being informed. Most leaflets are not very good, some are very poor, and some make no sense at all. One northern hospital produced a detailed leaflet on barium studies a few years ago that contained every known risk and complication, and details of preparation. However, it was soon noticed that patients still asked all the old questions. A journalist who was given one of these leaflets had a readability score calculated for it, and discovered that only the most intelligent 1% of the population could understand it. The moral here is that useful information presented in an inaccessible way is useless information. More recently, another northern hospital looked at consent forms for cataract patients and discovered that the print was so small that more than a third of the patients could not read the forms.

A standard hospital technique for obtaining informed consent is to throw information at the patient. The problem is that the information is standardised and the patient is unique – the information will mean different things to different patients depending on their health understanding, and what is readily understandable to one will be incomprehensible to another. A signature of consent may just mean that the patient trusts the doctors, not that they genuinely understand what is to be done to them and what risks there may be. Clinical trials are a really worrying area in this context, as patients tend to assume that any research that they enter into is safe. American research by the Hastings Center has shown that they do not read consent forms carefully because they assume that someone else has scrutinised the risks and benefits on their behalf. The main motive for enrolling was the belief that the experimental intervention was better than any existing alternative, and that it offered some personal benefit. Doctors' recommendations were, unsurprisingly, found to be very powerful factors influencing the decision to participate in trials. Many of the patients who were interviewed said that they had decided to take part before being given the consent form, and had then not bothered to read it. Doctors are still very influential people, and we must use this influence with care. We have previously mentioned our considerable dislike of the new verb 'to consent' – and sincerely hope that this is a communication strategy that withers on the vine.

Then there is the concept of implied consent – the patient rolling up the sleeve for a blood test, for example. This remains a difficult area. In extreme cases it is conceivable that doctors who treat without explicit consent may be breaching an individual's Article 8 rights (to a private life, free from interference) or even to Article 3 (the right not to be subjected to degrading treatment or torture) if side effects or consequences are severe. People who demand expensive life-extending drugs which are rationed due to the prohibitive cost and poor value for money may claim a breach of their right to life under Article 2. Obviously, where people lack capacity to consent the new Mental Capacity Act 2005 applies. This sets out statutory criteria for the test to be applied to determine whether someone can consent. Where people lack capacity according to these criteria treatment may be given in their best interests providing the reasoning is adequately set out. This is always a tricky area. The MCA enshrines the principle of an assumption of capacity. This suggests that we ought not to go looking too deeply for a lack of capacity where it is not obvious. However, many people probably understand considerably less than required to comprehend the treatments we propose. Then there is the issue of making unwise choices. People with capacity are allowed to make unwise or eccentric choices, but it is often very difficult to avoid seeing such decisions as de facto evidence of lack of capacity!

Here are a few statements from the NHS constitution of 2013 on this topic:

> No one can carry out any physical examination or give you treatment unless you have given your valid consent. You can therefore accept or refuse any treatment that is offered to you. If you lack capacity to consent yourself, and have given a person legal authority to make treatment decisions for you, then they can consent to or refuse treatment for you (this is called having a lasting power of attorney) where this would be in your best interests. If there is no such person then doctors will have to act in your best interests in deciding whether or not to carry out a treatment. Doctors must follow the guidance in the Mental Capacity Act when they make decisions in your best interest. . . . For children who are unable to consent to or refuse treatment because they lack sufficient understanding (i.e. they are not 'Gillick competent') parents may consent or refuse treatment where this would be in the child's best interests. . . . Investigation or treatment without valid consent may constitute a criminal offence or amount to battery. . . . Individual health professionals are also governed by the standards set under the professional regulatory regime that applies to their profession. You have the right to be given information about the test and treatment options available to you, what they involve and their risks and benefits. . . . When you are deciding whether to give your consent, this right entitles you to have the information you need to make a decision. The information you are given should include the benefits and the risks of the suggested treatment, as well as the risks if you decide not to take the suggested treatment. This information should be provided in a way that you can understand. Information about your treatment is an important part of your care and you should be given high quality information that is clear, accurate, impartial, balanced, evidence-based, easy to use and up-to-date . . .

It may be that informed consent is already an outmoded concept, and that instead patients should be encouraged to actively request a particular form of treatment after having been adequately informed of the options. This request shifts the onus on to the patient – the consumers of healthcare take responsibility for their choice. This is already happening in some settings, and the Government's patient choice initiative is fuelling the fire. This behaviour was unheard of when Peter wrote the first edition of this book in 1994. The availability of information from sources such as the Internet is speeding up this transition – our role as doctor is changing from informer to interpreter, so we need to get used to it. The future is now.

In many areas of healthcare, consent is taken for granted because the obvious benefit of the intervention obviates any dialogue. Much of the screening/prevention industry works on this premise. In fact it is often nothing more than a cycle of deceit and half-truths – consent is fudged because true understanding is not easy even for doctors, let alone patients. For example, consider regular breast self-examination, and start with the patient's point of view:

> Regular examination of my own breasts is a good idea because it will stop me from dying of breast cancer.

Well, the bad news is that it won't, or not on present evidence.

> If I find a lump it will mean I will stay healthy because I will have caught it in time.

This is not true, or if it is the difference is not great – operating on some lumps very early may even make the prognosis worse. Some lumps metastasise early and some don't – at present we cannot tell the difference.

> This must be a useful thing to do because the doctor/nurse/magazine told me to do it.

Really? The Chief Medical Officer did change his mind some years ago but was howled down and succumbed to encouraging breast awareness, whatever that is, instead.

> It stands to reason it must be a good idea.

It doesn't.

> It makes me worry about cancer, but prevention is better than cure, isn't it?

Not when the premise is a fallacy.
    Now try it from the doctor's point of view.

> It stands to reason it must be a good idea.

Have you looked long and hard at Wilson's criteria for screening recently?

> It cannot do any harm.

It can, not least in creating false expectations and contributing to the overvaluing of medical competence.

> I can't really tell her the truth – she wouldn't believe me.

It would take time, but she might. Honesty should be the best policy.

> But she will think I am an uncaring nihilist and that it does not worry me what happens to her.

If that is the case, you have not achieved any degree of shared understanding and it is still not worth perpetuating a dubious quarter-truth.

Try this exercise with cervical screening, cholesterol measurement, routine private medical screening, routine colonoscopies, screening for prostate cancer, etc., and ask yourself how much of the consent is really informed. There is a major ethical divide between your patient coming to you for your opinion and help with their agenda, and you imposing your screening agenda on that patient. If you do initiate such a procedure, you should have conclusive evidence that the test is likely to alter the outlook for that individual favourably, and that it is most unlikely to do any physical or psychological harm. You must face the issues honestly and help your patient to ask searching questions. At last the main body of the medical profession is waking up to this shameful state of affairs. The *British Medical Journal* produced a landmark edition in September 1999, entitled 'Embracing patient partnership' (it has a picture of a couple dancing the tango on the front cover).

Take the screening for bowel cancer using faecal occult blood (Smith *et al.*, 2010). In the published study they randomised those with a lower level of education into groups and in two groups they used decision support aids which clearly explained the procedure. The study revealed that those with more information reported that they knew more, made more informed choices and found the decision easier to make than those who did not receive further information. The surprising finding was that fewer of the educated group decided to take the test. The deeply depressing editorial accompanying this paper suggested that 'adherence' might be better achieved by 'a policy of informed uptake rather than informed decision making'.

A leading article by the sadly recently deceased Joan Austoker is a warning to the screening industry, and her final paragraph is worth quoting in full (Austoker, 1999):

Nevertheless, although uncertainties complicate the process of achieving informed consent, they underscore the importance of conducting research and taking care to ascertain what people believe about the disease and its causes, what they understand, and what they want to know. Ultimately informed patient choice, particularly about interventions that are both offered and delivered by health professionals, should take place in the context of shared decision making between the patient and health professional. Above all, we need to respect patients' autonomy – and that includes their right to decide not to undergo a screening intervention, even when refusal may result in harm to themselves.

The issue of screening for most patients is often that it is a necessary evil that is likely to confer health benefits. The possibility that screening may have harmful or negative effects is not often considered, but when faced by doctors communicating the results of screening there is much greater scepticism. In a study conducted in Australia, women patients carefully watched their doctor's non-verbal behaviour when they were receiving the results of their pap smear, in order to reach a conclusion about the doctor's veracity. The underlying issue was that of not trusting physicians to tell the whole truth.

In order to obtain true informed consent for cervical screening, doctors should:
- inform women of the limitations and disadvantages of the test
- inform women that the absolute benefit, to them as individuals, of their participation in the screening programme is extremely small
- inform women that as such screening accounts for part of the GP's income, there may be a conflict of interest
- check to ensure that women understand the issues
- read the General Medical Council's 1998 booklet *Seeking Patients' Consent: the ethical considerations.*

Consider the recent debate over mammography. According to an article by Jørgensen and Gøtzsche published in the *British Medical Journal* in 2009, doctors are likely to say that mammography will considerably improve the patient's chances of not dying of breast cancer. However, they are unlikely to say that if 2000 women are screened regularly for 10 years:
- 1 woman will benefit
- 10 healthy women will become cancer patients and undergo unnecessary treatment
- 200 women will experience a false alarm.

Several recent articles have shown increasingly conclusive evidence of harm from screening programmes, particularly prostate and breast cancer. Many agencies are calling for more screening, including for disorders such as dementia, but these should similarly be resisted until there is much clearer evidence of benefit.

The ethics of the doctor's agenda

This is a complex area that has received too little attention in the past. Again it relates to the implicit contract between doctor and patient, and the difficulties are most easily highlighted by a discussion of lifestyle advice and screening. Many doctors believe that the right to give unsolicited health and lifestyle advice is inherent in the nature of the relationship. The principle of beneficence comes into play – if the advice is for the patient's good it is ethically justified. Doctors who adhere strongly to such beliefs will view it as unethical to withhold such advice. Not all doctors would agree with this, and many find this a grey area, some developing an internalised scale of intrusiveness versus perceived benefit to the patient's health future. Some physicians who place patient autonomy high on their list of priorities will seldom offer such advice. Several authors, such as Illich, Skrabanek, McCormick and Iona Heath in her Pickles Lecture of 1999, have warned against any further unsolicited encroachments of medical advice into society, arguing about the dangers, the fallacies and the inherent uncertainty of widespread interference by doctors in the everyday lives of people in society.

To quote Heath (1999), an eminent GP working in Kentish Town, London, and one time president of the Royal College of General Practitioners:

> Medical science has valued the simple statistics of longevity above any measures of the quality of life. Many of our patients' palpable lack of enthusiasm for the 'lifestyle advice' we are obliged to deliver tells a different story, but the reordering of priorities is nonetheless both insidious and pernicious. . . . Much more work needs to be done to analyse and describe the limitations of biomedical science, the importance of death, and the overwhelming need to incorporate the patients' own values and aspirations into a system of care which is increasingly driven by standardised protocols. We must recognise the tendency for medical science to become totalitarian.

The insidious nature of this advice has been described as *coercive healthism.* The medical profession can easily slip into the role of the main arbiter of what is good for people, creating a climate of unjustified fear in an otherwise extremely healthy society. This whole (probably unstoppable) development is a major barrier to personal autonomy, is a continuation of the old beneficent paternalism, and there is a further danger of the doctor making negative value judgements when a conflict of health interests arises. A blaming culture arises, especially when doctors perceive that patients could do more to help themselves. Smoking and obesity often arouse strong victim-blaming reactions in doctors, producing unempathetic and often rather abrupt communication styles. The widespread rise in alcoholism and drug abuse has fuelled this difficulty, with many doctors stating that they will not treat such individuals, creating major difficulties in some emergency departments. The spread of AIDS has in some cases brought out the worst in the medical profession (as well as the best). These behaviours in patients, and developing the autonomy of the individual, pose major ethical problems for caring doctors – more so in organisations such as the NHS and managed care, where resources are clearly finite. Achieving a balance between beneficence, autonomy and justice is difficult. The communication imperative for the doctor should still be one of understanding. Issues of fairness, rationing and justice are better left outside the consulting room if at all possible.

The rise of the screening industry highlights this dilemma further. Health is seen as a commodity, immediately turning patients into consumers and consigning doctors to the role of middle managers in a health industry. New words are used. Old-style doctoring is replaced by 'anticipatory care', 'prevention' (which in this context only means a promise of a decreased likelihood of an event) and the now ubiquitous 'proactive' approach. As in Orwell's *1984*, language is used to conceal truth. The ethics of the relationship change dramatically. With good information the patient can decide on the risks and benefits of the procedure. If handled properly, this can lead to acceptable informed consent and an ethically defensible contract, but as already stated many of the existing screening programmes short-circuit the consent issue. Some are even deliberately economical with the truth, emphasising the benefits while playing down the uncertainties, risks and detrimental effects. Again, apologists will cite the beneficent arguments while playing down autonomy.

Western societies are increasingly concerned about health, para-doxically at a time when it has never been better. Individual patients vary with regard to their own personal concern. Some people have always had an unhealthy obsession with health, as Mark Twain pointed out:

> There are people who strictly deprive themselves of each and every eatable, drinkable and smokeable which has in any way acquired a shady reputation. They pay this price for health. And health is all they get out of it. It is like paying out your whole fortune for a cow that has gone dry.

Patients for whom personal health, prevention, well-being and longevity are high on their agenda are also invoking their right to be heard. This can pose problems in predominantly disease- and problem-based systems of care. Conflicts of agenda can arise, autonomy coming into conflict with justice in the form of time rationing. The place of these issues in the primary care consultation and outpatient meeting remains unresolved.

One of our difficulties is that our agenda as doctors is being constantly expanded, with uncertain consequences for patients. The cholesterol debate illustrates this increasing nightmare. As we write it is now agreed that secondary prevention of heart disease by lowering cholesterol is a good and evidence-based strategy for our population. This means that all patients with any suggestion of heart trouble come under the umbrella of medical care for the rest of their lives. Fair enough, you say, and you might be right. The next step, suggested by trials on high-risk but healthy men in the West of Scotland, is that most of us should take cholesterol-lowering drugs for the rest of our lives. Apart from the horrendous cost to the Exchequer, this means that most of the adult population will become patients. A sliver of sense is visible across the wide Atlantic. There is new guidance on cholesterol from the US (late 2013) which suggests that aggressively targeting cholesterol concentration should be abandoned in favour of an approach which targets overall cardiovascular risk. While this does remove those arbitrary cholesterol thresholds, it strikes us that this will have little practical impact, as most doctors will still be faced with people with high risk who can't or won't make significant life-style changes themselves. They are then still faced with the prospect of medicalising them in order to theoretically reduce the likelihood of cardiovascular events. Quite how most patients are expected to consent to this is anyone's guess.

We are now bombarded by frightening-looking journals full of statistics about the numbers of people who need to be treated for so many years in order to prevent some event. We still do not know how this really helps us to treat worried Mr Hay sitting nervously clutching and unclutching his umbrella in outpatients. We do know that we are both going to die of something, and that our job as his doctor is to help him to live as healthy a life as possible in the context of our society. We shall all need to be informed on this debate, have our cholesterol monitored and increase the burden on the health industry. It seems that Ivan Illich is right, and that we are increasingly medicalising all aspects of our lives. This worries us. Does it worry you?

Hypertension – as we said in Chapter 4, a doctor's disease if ever there was one – has now reached plague proportions. Depending on which set of guidelines you use, over 50% of over-75s should be on active treatment. If you stand back from this thought for a second, you begin to wonder if the lunatics are taking over the asylum. Let us remind you that this is not a benign diagnosis. Irrespective of treatment, the diagnosis is associated with an 80% increase in absenteeism, sport is avoided, impotence rates quadruple, and the 'hypertensive' person now sees himself or herself differently. They become preoccupied with sickness and their energy levels decline. In one study using the Quality of Life Impairment Scale, 30% of patients classified themselves as 'severely ill'. This is a label that makes people sick, so we doctors have to do an awful lot of good to make up for it. David Misselbrook, in his excellent book *Thinking about Patients* (2001), suggests that you ask all of your hypertensive patients three questions:

1 Do you ever wonder if you might be experiencing side effects from your medication?
2 Do you often think about your blood pressure?
3 Does your blood pressure cause you any problems in your day-to-day life?

He found very high levels of anxiety and a feeling of being stigmatised by the label. Try it yourself.

The real crux of the whole informed consent debate is that to obtain true informed consent requires the achievement of a *shared understanding and a shared management plan.* This further implies that the patient's beliefs should be known and their understanding checked effectively. The ethical imperative behind achieving a shared understanding is respect for the individual. To achieve these tasks at all requires a belief by the physician that sharing with patients is a desirable outcome. This is not and never can be a framework for paternalistic consulting. Ethically, this has to be a true belief, not a Machiavellian means of achieving the outcome desired by the doctor. Most doctors are not that pure and, while espousing the patient-centred method, will use it to manipulate the patient in a beneficent but paternalistic way.

There is an assumption that consent can never be truly informed, so that it is for doctors to determine what is in the patient's best interest. However, health is mainly the subjective experience of an individual and is made up of highly personal beliefs, feelings and experiences. It follows that, when helped by physicians to achieve a comprehension of the risks and benefits of various treatments, it is patients and only patients who can really determine which therapy will help them to achieve their most important health goals.

It has always seemed to us that one of the ethical hallmarks of good medical communication is a requirement for honesty. There is an imperative for the doctor to seek and confirm understanding in four main areas: first, that the patient is aware that they are an active part of the decision-making process; second, that they are aware of the choices; third, that they are aware of the implications of those choices; and, finally, that they have assimilated enough specific information on the risks and benefits to allow them to make an informed choice. Sadly, although this may be the ideal ethical position, recordings of consultations of young doctors suggest that such behaviour is by no means the norm.

The communication of risk–benefit advice is an interesting area. This is communication at its most difficult, and in this age of evidence-based choice doctors will need to learn to do it well. Patients who are well informed will often make choices of which doctors may not approve. The medical benefits of stroke prevention by warfarin in atrial fibrillation seem to be clear, but in a group of patients who were well informed of the risks and benefits, a significant proportion decided not to choose the intervention. Several studies have demonstrated that the method of communicating risk significantly affects patient uptake. Numbers needed to treat patients with mild hypertension in order to prevent one event provide a very different perspective to saying that taking a particular intervention halves an already small risk. This is an area where 'framing' the questions can easily distort the truth, whatever that is – 'spin' is a more popular word for the same idea.

For example, most doctors are likely to tell patients that trials show that treatment is indicated for mild hypertension, and that treatment will prevent them from having a stroke. They won't usually say that there is a 99.8% probability that treatment will do the individual no good in any given year, that treatment fails to prevent the majority of strokes, and that the very marginal benefits of treatment need to be set against the anxiety, medicalisation, side effects and expense of treatment. The scope for unethical and manipulative behaviour is very wide, often fuelled by the profit-related motives of pharmaceutical companies.

The truth is that patients need a certain understanding of basic statistics to understand even the simple medical messages. Sadly, our educational system does not seem to be up to this task and very few of our patients have any real grasp of the issues at stake.

> Understanding risks and asking critical questions can also shape the emotional climate in a society, so that hopes and anxieties are no longer as easily manipulated from outside and citizens can develop a better informed and more relaxed attitude toward their health.
>
> Gigerenzer *et al.* (2008)

The major problem with risk is the differing frames of reference used by patients and doctors. Doctors use mathematical concepts, absolute risk, relative risk and numbers needed to treat. Patients with varying loci of control see themselves, for very unmathematical reasons, as being high, medium or low risk, and then use the lottery logic of luck, fate and destiny to make an individual and unique assessment. If we let them, our patients will tell us compelling stories to communicate their perceptions to us, having already swapped stories in the pub in order to construct their own sense of reality. We doctors, on the other hand, relate statistics but without the persuasive reality and impact of the stories that our patients relate. It means that doctors could do worse than learn to relate counter-stories to combat our patients' tales

– this is high-level communication and is likely to be unusual. The burning unanswerable question that our patient wants to ask is 'Do you really think that taking this tablet for the next 30 years is definitely going to do me more good than harm?' We don't know if you back horses, but most gamblers wouldn't touch the odds for 'treating' mild hypertension. Interestingly, numbers needed to treat (NNTs) are quite difficult to find at present. In fact it has got worse since the 2007 edition! Even with the Internet, it is not easy. You should read an article entitled 'Communicating risks: illusion or truth?' published in a themed issue of the *British Medical Journal* in September 2003.

Patient utilities is an expression that has been gaining ground since the earlier editions of this book. It is a rather inelegant American way of defining what matters to patients. This has allowed us to rethink some older but interesting measures, such as von Neumann's 'Standard Gamble', which balances the negative utility of a particular outcome against a risk of sudden death, and tries to define what risk an individual is actually prepared to take. Another is Torrance's 'Time Trade-Off', which defines the value of improvements in health by a comparison with the life expectancy that an individual is prepared to forgo in order to achieve them. Misselbrook again advocates a new measure, which is the inverse of NNTs, that he calls the 'Personal Probability of Benefit' (PPB), and he goes on to argue that if we do not explain the low probability of benefit to patients there can be no informed consent.

When trying to achieve shared decision making, it is permissible – perhaps even morally obligatory – for a doctor to attempt by negotiation to change the mind of a patient who is making an apparently silly or irrational choice. It is through these genuine negotiations that the doctor and patient can come to a truly shared understanding of the issues in a way that is best suited to maximising the values of both. However, although the decision-making process is shared, the final decision is that of the patient. It has to be said, though, that it must be correct, in extreme cases of conflict of belief, for physicians to retain the power not to treat patients if the management choice and plan require them to act in a manner that they believe is unethical. By its very nature negotiating with a patient may result in an outcome you are unsatisfied with. While patients cannot demand we prescribe something we believe to be wholly inappropriate, there is usually a much greyer area where we are persuaded to up a dose or prescribe something which just might help but we don't honestly believe actually will. The ethics of this, not to mention the view of the GMC and NICE on this, are debatable. Effective communication in this instance may have been achieved, but at what cost? Hopefully, not to our own professional registration and probably most judgements would still be upheld by a jury of our peers.

A good model must be one of *mutual persuasion* by two experts, one on medical matters and the other on their own mind and body. This implies that doctors must be prepared to allow themselves to be persuaded by their patients away from their first or second choices of action if the patient's argument is effective, convincing and – most importantly – informed. Doctors are not always going to like this.

Any doctor who wants to be effective must be interested in people and not merely diseases. They must be committed to their patients' welfare, willing to search out their patients' beliefs, and it follows that they must also be willing to listen to whatever problems the patients bring to them. This is an intensely personal form of doctoring, which is not seen in modern hospitals very often. The treatment of a disease can be largely impersonal, but the care of a patient is entirely personal.

Patients in the UK are now entitled to see your thinking, or at least that which you commit to paper, again to quote the NHS constitution of 2013:

> Patients can ask for, and should receive, copies of letters and other correspondence about their care. This includes letters on referral, letters following outpatient appointments and discharge letters that are sent routinely between clinicians as part of patient care.

The General Medical Council (2000), in its *Duties of a Doctor*, is unequivocal in its position on the duties of a doctor:

> Patients must be able to trust doctors with their lives and well-being. To justify that trust, we as a profession have a duty to maintain a good standard of practice and care and to show respect for human life. In particular, as a doctor you must:
> - make the care of your patient your first concern
> - treat every patient politely and considerately
> - respect patients' dignity and privacy
> - listen to patients and respect their views

- give patients information in a form that they can understand
- respect the right of patients to be fully involved in decisions about their care
- keep your professional knowledge and skills up to date
- recognise the limits of your professional competence
- be honest and trustworthy
- respect and protect confidential information
- make sure that your personal beliefs do not prejudice your patients' care
- act quickly to protect patients from risk if you have good reason to believe that you or a colleague may not be fit to practise
- avoid abusing your position as a doctor
- work with colleagues in the ways that best serve patients' interests.

In all of these matters you must never discriminate unfairly against your patients or colleagues. And you must always be prepared to justify your actions to them.

References

Austoker J. Gaining informed consent for screening is difficult – but many misconceptions need to be undone. *BMJ*. 1999; **319**: 722–3.

Communicating risks: illusion or truth? *BMJ*. 2003; **327**(7417).

Department of Health. *NHS Constitution*. London: Department of Health; 2013.

Embracing patient partnership. *BMJ*. 1999; **319**(7212).

Fowler FJ Jr, Gerstein BS, Barry MJ. How patient centered are medical decisions? Results of a national survey. *BMJ*. 173(13): 1215–21.

General Medical Council. *Duties of a Doctor*. London: General Medical Council; 2000.

General Medical Council. *Seeking Patients' Consent: the ethical considerations*. London: General Medical Council; 1998.

Gigerenzer GW, Gaissmaier W, Kurz-Milcke E, *et al*. Helping doctors and patients make sense of health statistics. *Psychol Sci Public Interest*. 2008; 8(2): 53–96.

Greenfield S, Kaplan S, Ware JE Jr. Expanding patient involvement in care: effects on patient outcomes. *Ann Intern Med*. 1985; **102**(4): 520–8.

Heath I. William Pickles Lecture 1999: 'Uncertain clarity': contradiction, meaning, and hope. *Br J Gen Pract*. 1999; **49**(445): 651–7.

Illich I. *Medical Nemesis*. London: Marion Boyars; 1975.

Illman J, Kirkness B, Association of British Pharmaceutical Industry. *The Expert Patient*. London: Association of the British Pharmaceutical Association; 2000.

Jørgensen KJ, Gøtzsche PC. Overdiagnosis in publicly organised mammography screening programmes: systematic review of incidence trends. *BMJ*. 2009; **339**: b2587.

Misselbrook D. *Thinking about Patients*. Newbury: Petroc Press; 2001.

Mulley AG, Trimble C, Elwyn G. Stop the silent misdiagnosis: patients' preferences matter. *BMJ*. 2012; **345**: e6572.

Smith SK, Trevena L, Simpson JM *et al*. A decision aid to support informed choices about bowel cancer screening among adults with low education: randomised controlled trial. *BMJ*. 2010; **341**: c5370.

CHAPTER 11

The essence of good doctoring: a personal interlude

> *The patient will never care how much you know until they know how much you care.*
>
> Terry Canale, American Academy of Orthopaedic Surgeons
> Vice Presidential Address (Tongue *et al.*, 2005)

Peter's reflection on his medical career

How should we distil the essence of good doctoring? What are the precious formulas that we would want to pass on to the next generation? What must we preserve and are there any babies we can let slip with the bath water?

Has the essence changed much over the years? I can help you there. I can tell you about my father who was a GP in South Shields, on the Tyne. He was already there when Aneurin Bevin imposed the NHS on an extremely unwilling profession in 1948. He hated the NHS all his life, perceiving it as patronising, Stalinist and restrictive. He did love his patients, and was lucky to love his job. I say lucky because the job was perhaps even more all pervasive than it is today. As a single-hander, as most were, the 24-hour commitment was real, locums were scarce and expensive, and deputising was unheard of. His surgery was in a basement in Beach Road, with peeling wallpaper, a smell of damp, and 'The Monarch of the Glen' on the wall. My mother was the receptionist, nurse, dragon and saint at the gate. There were no appointment systems, no team meetings, no special clinics, no computers, and to be honest no notes worth the candle. There was a lot of work. 'The Surgery' started at 8.15, and ended 40 or so patients later at around 11 am. There were then 10-plus visits and another 'surgery' between 4 and 7 pm, often with a couple more visits on the way home, and most evenings disturbed by more phone calls and other visits. Telephone advice was not considered quite proper then.

The work was unfiltered, haphazard and very popular – sick notes, ear syringing, boil lancing, home births, general advice, drastic pharmacology such as barbiturates, amphetamines, methyldopa, personally mixed placebos, and the green, red and black bottle.

My father kept going until 1975, and died suddenly of a mixture of heart disease, a very unhealthy lifestyle and myasthenia gravis. He was 58 and still single-handed.

I came up from the south to help my mother to clear out his surgery. The old microscope, the pestle and mortar, the empty gin bottles, and about 5 years of *BMJ* issues, still in their brown wrappers, were piled up on the examination couch. Dad's desk was a big one, and the patient's chair was tatty and rickety, placed directly in front.

His funeral at the local crematorium was attended by a larger crowd than the average Sunderland AFC match. So many people I didn't know came up to embrace me (a rare thing for Geordies) and said how much they loved him, but one man stands out in my mind. He sought me out as the crowd was dispersing. He held my hand and looked at me hard.

'Peter, isn't it? And you a doctor, too. Not as good as him, though. Your dad, he was special. He used to listen to you. Didn't examine you much.' I had worked that one out.

'But he listened, and he knew. He always knew, never wrong, because he always listened he always knew what mattered.'

I qualified from Newcastle in 1968, 46 years ago, and then ran away to sea and spent a couple of years as senior surgeon with P&O. This was old-fashioned general practice – no continuity, though – but you did whatever needed doing. Great stuff. In 1972 I became a trainee in Kentish Town with John Horder and Mike Modell. A slightly different breed from my father, they were more overtly academic, less steeped in the day-to-day and more visionary. They were members of the Royal College of General Practitioners and – most different of all – worked in a group, a health centre, almost a polyclinic. Here I met professionals I had never encountered before, such as health visitors, social workers, mental health officers, community psychiatrists, practice nurses and practice managers, and there were wonderful things like night rotas and embryonic deputising systems.

My overwhelming memory of that time is enthusiasm for general practice. Snotty little toad that I was, I wrote to my trainers at the end of the year and highlighted the three areas in which they had most improved my ability to help people. These were:
- listening properly to what patients say
- using time as a diagnostic tool and as a method of understanding people better
- good note keeping – I described this as the root from which all else flows, and I can hear my partners' hollow laughter in my ear.

I took a partnership in Abingdon-on-Thames in 1973 and lasted 30 years there, until the coronary arteries malfunctioned. I was promoted beyond the level of my own competence in 1978 to be the Oxford District GP course organiser, but I was not sure what to teach. I did not really know what I knew, and I was not yet entirely clear what the secret of good doctoring really was. I was aware that it had something to do with communication. I had also read learned treatises on knowledge, skills and attitudes, and had tried to digest my trainers' *The Future General Practitioner: learning and teaching*. However, it was all rather a blur in my mind. Then I met David Pendleton, retired evangelist turned social psychologist, who had come to Oxford to seek answers about the relationship between doctors and patients. We became friends, and I took a sabbatical and went to work with him in the Department of Experimental Psychology. This place was awash with frighteningly clever people, who were at this time mostly into attribution theory, or why people do what they do.

David had read Pat Byrne and Barrie Long's *Doctors Talking to Patients* (1976), based on research in which they had audiotaped more than 2000 consultations. We had an early Sony black-and-white video camera, so we started getting our GP friends, trainers and course organisers to videotape some consultations, and we began to analyse them, looking for the substance, the kernel, the essence. David interviewed the patients before and afterwards, and found that their views of the consultation were not the same as those of the doctor, and often differed markedly from them. Misunderstanding was the norm. Theo Schofield, Peter Havelock, David and I were working closely together by this stage, and we felt that the consultation between doctor and patient needed to be demystified and the essential tasks clearly delineated. We did this, and out of attribution theory and the health belief model came ICE, a mnemonic that has spawned a thousand courses, and we stated that the real essence of any consultation was for both parties to achieve as genuine a shared understanding as possible.

This, as you know, is a difficult thing to do.

The Consultation: an approach to learning and teaching was published in 1984 by Oxford University Press. Ten years later, frustrated by the relative lack of progress in persuading others of the goal of shared understanding, a group of enthusiasts, including Roger Neighbour, Peter Campion, Lesley Southgate and Steve Field, helped by the genius of John Foulkes, began to introduce the video examination into the MRCGP. This was an unashamed attempt to influence the teaching curriculum to move good consulting up the ladder of importance. In 1994 I wrote the first edition of this, *The Doctor's Communication Handbook*, which was intended to be a user-friendly manual for the new examination. The video examination has now come and gone, and *The Doctor's Communication Handbook* is in its seventh edition and has a new author, but the goal of a shared understanding remains.

What all those thousands of videotapes of young doctors demonstrated most clearly was the very special relationship that patients have with doctors. This represents a continuity in our society that has existed from the shamans to the present day. A fundamental component of that relationship is trust, which can be cemented by the smallest degree of personal continuity and demonstrated caritas.

I will let you into an embarrassing secret. I like old Westerns. One of my favourites is John Ford's *Stagecoach* (at least I am in good company there, as Orson Welles is said to have watched it over 100 times before making *Citizen Kane*). One of the beguiling aspects of the film is the behaviour of the doctor. We meet him debt-ridden, fleeing town and hopelessly addicted to whisky. We learn that his addiction may be related to the unspeakable horrors he has witnessed in the Civil War, and that he has abandoned all pretence of professionalism and sobriety. He insinuates himself shamelessly with a mouse of a whisky salesman, and as the stagecoach rolls along through Indian country he drinks the poor man's wares. Then of course comes the dramatic twist – the young cavalry officer's wife goes into labour at a stage halt, and medical skills, as well as plenty of hot water, are called for. In one of the subplots the socially despised 'tart with a heart' has to act as midwife to the upper-class lady. The doctor sobers up dramatically with the help of plenty of hot coffee, and proceeds to perform the necessary medical duties through a difficult but successful birth. So far so clichéd, but good nonetheless. However, it is the scene after the birth that is most revealing. In the dark semiotic corridor, the prostitute pours out her problems to the doctor. Should she go away with the handsome young Ringo (played, of course, by John Wayne)? Should she tell him 'the sort of girl she is'? Could the doctor stop him going to a showdown where he will almost certainly be killed?

The point about these questions and requests that she directs at the newly rehabilitated doctor is that none of them is remotely medical. He is bemused but kindly and does his best, but why does she ask him these deeply personal questions? Of course it is because she trusts him, and that is because he has just proved himself, despite all of his past failings, as worthy of that trust.

You are going to be trusted, whether you like it or not. You must consider this, as it is very important (*see* Figure 11.1).

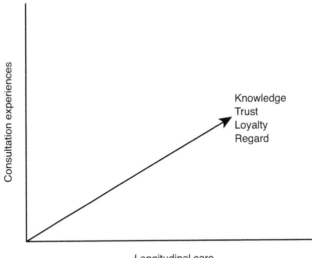

FIGURE 11.1 Trust and time (Ridd *et al.*, 2009)

What British doctors possess, almost uniquely, is a relative freedom from financial pressures. Our opinions are almost unbiased and our patients know that. This is something worth fighting for – retaining our patients' trust.

What we learned from the 10-year video experiment was that good consulting is not a natural gift for most of us. It has to be worked at, it has to be practised and it has to be critiqued.

If the generalist is to have a unique place in twenty-first-century medicine, it must surely be as the last outpost of personal medicine. 'Personal' means tailored to the individual. This means involving the individual and finding out what matters to them, and it means good consulting, which is not easy, as over 10 years of video examinations have conclusively proved. We are also entering an era of organised discontinuity. We must try to resist this powerful trend, but we must also realise the main implication of this break-up of the traditional relationship. It means that you will have to communicate more effectively than me, as you may not get the second chance that my father and I relied upon.

To remind you again, after 5000 years the role of the doctor has changed. You are no longer the keepers of occult truths and mysteries – the Internet has seen to that. Instead you will be the interpreters of health-related information. Not all of you will have realised that this will be your major role in this still young century. To fulfil this role you will need knowledge, medical expertise and good organisations, but more than that you must be driven by internal needs that will help you to help your patients in an ever changing world.

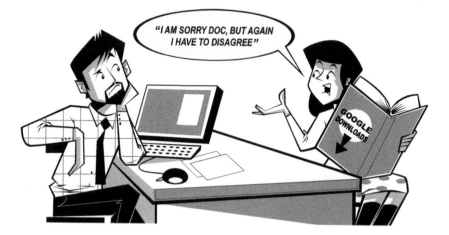

You will need to fight to retain your relationships with patients, where your very presence raises hopes and offers a little magic, and perhaps the more you are known the more your patients may derive succour from just knowing you. Therapeutically, you become a very small sea wall between them and the vast ocean of life.

So what are these internal drivers that lead us to the very essence of your job? There are three of them, I think.

First and perhaps most important is *curiosity* – a desire to discover what really matters to your patient. This leads, secondly, to a need to help your patients to *understand*, which leads, thirdly, to an understanding of *trust*. Trust is there, whether you seek it or not, so perhaps it should drive you. These three drivers were important to my father, and helped me through my own career, and perhaps they will help you in yours.

Both my father and I qualified from Durham/Newcastle University. My father knew and told me of the great Geordie paediatrician Sir James Spence commemorated at the Royal Victoria Infirmary to this day. His most famous quotation is as follows:

> The real work of a doctor is not an affair of health centres, or laboratories, or hospital beds. Techniques have their place in medicine, but they are not medicine. The essential unit of medical practice is the occasion when, in the intimacy of the consulting room or sick room, a person who is ill, or believes himself to be ill, seeks the advice of a doctor whom he trusts. This is a consultation, and all else in the practice of medicine derives from it.
>
> (1938)

I have lived my whole career with that quote echoing in my brain, but Liz has made me aware that the word 'consultation' is in decline in primary care and has virtually disappeared from hospital medicine, and even more worrying to me nothing has replaced it. To make this little guide acceptable to young doctors in hospital we have removed nearly all references to the 'consultation' and substituted 'communication' or similar. This is a shame; it is a lessening of the meaning, an involuntary demeaning of the relationship and a loss of trust. Think of an embracing new word or bring it back, please.

References

Byrne PS, Long BEL. *Doctors Talking to Patients: a study of the verbal behaviours of doctors in the consultation*. London: Her Majesty's Stationery Office; 1976.

Horder JP, Byrne PS, Freeling P, *et al. The Future General Practitioner: learning and teaching*. London: The Royal College of General Practitioners; 1972.

Pendleton D, Schofield T, Tate P, *et al. The Consultation: an approach to learning and teaching*. Oxford: Oxford University Press; 1984.

Ridd M, Shaw A, Lewis G, *et al.* The patient–doctor relationship: a synthesis of the qualitative literature on patients' perspectives. *Br J Gen Pract.* 2009; 59: 268–75.

Tongue JR, Epps HR, Forese LL. Communication skills for patient-centered care: research-based, easily learned techniques for medical interviews that benefit orthopaedic surgeons and their patients. *J Bone Joint Surg Am.* 2005; 87: 652–8.

CHAPTER 12

Communication as a competence?

Communication – the key to avoiding catastrophe

> *The single biggest problem in communication is the illusion that it has taken place.*

George Bernard Shaw

Countless enquiries and critical incident reviews have consistently demonstrated the fact that failures in communication account for more complaints and errors than any other single factor in medicine. The recent high-profile Francis Report identified failures in communication as one of the single most significant factors in the abject failure of care at Mid Staffordshire. Perhaps more than ever before communication is being recognised as a key skill in every medical speciality. Maybe even *the* key skill. Communication skills and 'human factor' courses abound. The terminology is certainly ubiquitous in every area of medicine now, but there remains considerable confusion and inconsistency in expectation and assessment. Put simply, every doctor is told regularly that they have to communicate effectively, but few get any actual guidance on what this looks like in real life, or how to actually do it themselves.

Some of us wrongly assume that having got to this stage in our career we must be doing it right. Similarly, little external scrutiny is made of doctors once they have completed their training as they are presumed to have all the requisite competencies, including excellent communication skills. Doctors typically get little or no feedback on their interactions with patients either from their patients or from their colleagues and consequently are rarely confronted by their shortcomings. Feedback on our performance is something we must actively seek and for many this is just too terrifying. Some doctors have embraced the use of technology for this purpose and invite their patients to review and rate their performance on various doctor comparison websites. While laudable for promoting transparency, it remains to be seen whether this form of feedback is actually helpful or translates into real changes in behaviour.

Evidence

Demonstrating effective communication with patients and relatives is a requirement in every speciality training curriculum and every single doctor must now provide evidence of their ability to communicate effectively in order to revalidate. 'Good communication skills' is seen by many as the Holy Grail of workplace-based assessments, which are increasingly the mechanism by which trainee doctors are assessed. However, many doctors give very little consideration to what their communication tasks actually are, what skills they need, or what they look like and few really know how to recognise them in practice. A nice manner (the 'common nice mumble') is probably substituted in many instances. This may be the halo effect in action – if the doctor appears to be nice the assessor will assume they are doing a good job of communicating.

Curriculums

Most doctors in training never read their curriculum and if they do typically find it an impenetrable document which seems to bear scant relation to the job they do or the skills they believe they must master. The General Adult Psychiatry one alone is a complex matrix some 156 pages long. Whatever your speciality, however, 'communication' is guaranteed to be in there somewhere. The small minority who get as far as reading their own curriculum will probably skip the section on communication entirely, perhaps assuming that their communication skills are already satisfactory, or maybe realising that it is very easy to produce 'evidence' of communication skills and very difficult for anyone to prove that your abilities in this area are inadequate.

The role of the trainer?

Whose responsibility is it to ensure that you communicate well? The GMC would assert that it is yours as the doctor, and ensuring you master this skill is part of your professional responsibility. However, if you are on a training scheme maybe you would argue it is the responsibility of whichever organisation provides and organises your programme. After all, deaneries and health education boards are paid to train a competent doctor – does this include ensuring the doctor can communicate effectively? Should they offer the training and invite doctors to participate if they consider their particular skill-set requires it, or should this be mandatory? Perhaps it should be the role of your educational supervisor to assess and develop your communication skills? This may be true in general practice, where this skill is possibly still more highly valued and the structure of training often lends itself to this kind of development. However, it would probably seem laughable to many hospital doctors to expect their consultants to give them pointers on talking to patients more effectively.

The good news (for you) is of course that the very fact you are reading this book indicates you have an insight into your own practice and an open-mindedness about developing your own repertoire of skills. Doctors who are very poor communicators rarely realise this fact and few seek help. For many people it is still highly humiliating and stigmatising to accept a problem in this fundamental area. After all, talking and listening can't be that hard, right? Of course, doctors who are unconsciously incompetent will never take steps to improve as they remain unaware of their weakness. Even doctors who are consciously incompetent may be deterred from seeking help; for example, to overcome language problems. Obviously, we cannot be perfect communicators all the time. Some interactions are harder than others and sometimes all the skills in our toolkit will not be enough. To appropriate DW Winnicott's (a famous psychoanalytic paediatrician) principle of the 'good-enough' mother, perhaps to achieve enough competence to be a 'good-enough' communicator is a reasonable aspiration?

Assessing communication

Communication is a component of every structured workplace-based assessment. Designed ostensibly to be a formative instrument, these are still widely used as a summative form of assessment with scores given according to the perceived performance. A certain number of these are required for every doctor in training in order to pass their annual appraisal or ARCP. The usefulness of these assessments varies widely and even doctors who value them as a learning exercise may not actually learn much from them. Relief at getting a good score is likely to result in dismissal of any development points, while poor scores typically result in inaction due to a sense of injustice and help-lessness. Doctors are often assessed by colleagues who themselves have no understanding of the expected criteria for that particular doctor's level of experience and are unfamiliar with the instruments.

Exactly how the communication skills of an F2 differ from those expected of an ST6 is one question which is never satisfactorily defined. Perhaps all of us are expected to have consultant-level com-munication skills from day one of our careers? If there is a gradation of expectation, how exactly do we quantify and manage this? What about the person who consistently passes their ARCP but everyone knows they can't communicate for toffee, make errors as a result, and often leave their patients in tears? Conversely, a minority of trainees do fail their ARCPs and their professional exams, and training organi-sations are often left unsure how to help them. Undoubtedly, the most common reason for failure to progress is inadequate communication skills.

No one has yet clearly identified the magic ingredient that sepa-rates the novice from the expert in medicine. Observing many doctors consulting both well and badly suggests that a good knowledge base and a willingness to listen and act on what the patient tells you is a good start, but not sufficient. Experience can work both ways: if it shuts down the search too quickly it is unhelpful; if it allows explora-tion of paths not easily seen it is useful. A simple guide to effective or less effective problem solving is the time to the examination in a new problem. In most cases, the physical examination signals the end of the problem-solving phase, the examination is usually confirmatory, very seldom revelatory and the explanation that follows is already etched in stone. So a very simple heuristic: the quicker the examin-ation, the more fragile the problem solving. With complex problems it is of course even more difficult; the most helpful skill in these cases is the ability to remain open to new ideas and information. The effective synthesis of all this information is what separates the diffident novice from the true expert, and the fact that some are better than others at this suggests that it is a subtle mix of the 'science' of clinical reasoning and the 'art' of good medical practice.

Most doctors add to their factual knowledge cumulatively and as they practise applying that knowledge, a deeper understanding develops. As their knowledge and problem-solving skill improve within a domain, problem-solving behaviours become more 'expert-like'. We do really have to emphasise the positive – yes, we make mistakes but expert clinical reasoning is very likely to be right in the majority of cases.

When it comes to exams, communication is increasingly assessed through direct observation of doctors in standardised simulated situations. Serious questions continue to be raised about the validity of this system, although the practical advantages compared to the old vivas and long cases are undeniable. Assessment of communication competence relies on establishing what the measurable goals of the interaction are. Concepts such as 'establishes rapport', 'puts patient at ease' and 'introduces self' are accepted, although rarely examined beyond the superficial. It seems for those who find this easy there is no need for examination and for those who find it difficult there is little practical formative help available. Similarly, 'demonstrates empathy' is a concept some doctors find very difficult. Perhaps those who find this easy to demonstrate are particularly good at seeing things from the patient's perspective or maybe they are just better at faking?

Criteria can help, but agreeing them in the first place and then recognising what was agreed is not easy. Just think about the task: 'Dr picks up cues'. There is almost total agreement that this seems a necessary criterion to demonstrate competence in the medical encounter, but there is very little agreement among experienced assessors about what this apparently simple and unequivocal statement actually means.

Training vs education

Competency-based training is in vogue right now. The apprenticeship model is seen as old-fashioned. Organisations want measurable nuggets of skill, preferably squeezed into as short a training programme as possible that delivers the best possible value for money. Doctors rarely work exclusively with a single 'firm' attached to a single consultant any more. Many juniors go straight from medical school into unbanded posts (9 to 5 with no on-call commitment). Fewer hours at work mean fewer hours of acquiring exposure to medicine, and this has fuelled the targeted skills-based training explosion. Training schemes understandably want to offer standardised training that produces measurable outcomes. However, communication as a unit of competence is trickier. While essential tasks in the doctor–patient interaction have been identified and can arguably be measured, it is much more subjective. Attempting to determine whether Dr A adequately elicited Mr Gale's real concerns and fears about his chest pain is inevitably much more difficult compared with agreeing whether Dr A was able to adequately site a Venflon. Training courses for communication are consequently much more difficult to pitch and fund. Even when everyone agrees that communication is essential, without easy measurable outcomes from such interventions few hospitals and training schemes prioritise it. Breaking communication down into achievable tasks or framing it as an essential skill (such as 'breaking bad news') does help.

Communication is something everyone does!

Increasingly, patients are assessed and followed up by other health professionals and this outsourcing of medical wisdom, while possibly good for patients in many instances, may have inadvertently devalued the importance of doctor–patient communication. Other professionals can apparently do it without any of the navel gazing required of doctors, so it can't be that hard, right? They don't have to attend communication skills training sessions or produce evidence of it in their portfolios. If the key unit of the medical consultation was communication and other allied health professionals can now do this as well as we can, then what exactly is our role again? This may be one of the reasons why psychiatry is experiencing an acute loss of identity – the central skill (that of the doctor–patient therapeutic interaction) is increasingly done by other members of the team, relegating the doctor's role to one of prescription and rubber-stamping.

Perhaps these other professionals have been able to retain their natural empathy and skill in talking to people which, historically, medical school drummed out of young doctors? Or maybe they aren't very good communicators either and more needs to be done to ensure the value of this essential skill is recognised all round. Interestingly, a number of critical incident reviews in recent years concluded that removing doctors from the central leadership role in clinical teams was directly responsible for catastrophic failures of care, and they recommended that they be reinstated, so we must be doing something right.

Good communicator, bad doctor?

Of course it is possible to be a good communicator, at least in the sense of being especially empathetic and developing a superb rapport and therapeutic relationship, but still be a poor doctor. After all, Harold Shipman was supposedly widely liked by his patients. Communication is just one of the many skills required of a doctor. It's almost impossible to be any good without it, but you can still be bad even if you do it well. Applied knowledge, pattern recognition, decision making and situational judgement are just a few other skills without which good communication remains just being nice to people. And patients can get that elsewhere. The task remains central. How many doctors really ask themselves what this is?

The hardest task for all doctors is learning to cope with the essential uncertainty and unpredictability of illness. This requires a humility not always fostered in certain training schemes. Communication with our patients in such an uncertain world is quite difficult. Doctors are trained in probability, and those of an authoritarian bent prefer telling to listening, and can easily slip into a well-intentioned but malignant form of paternalistic dishonesty. This is both poor communication and bad medicine. You will have to learn to share uncertainty and avoid pretending that you know everything. You will not always be popular.

Motivation

This is probably the key to it all. We won't communicate well with patients or anyone else if we lack the motivation to do so. Exams are an excellent motivator, of course. They are not only essential to our progression but they are inordinately expensive, which only increases the drive to pass first time. If communication must be demonstrated to pass we learn how to do it, even if it does not come naturally to us.

Once they are over, however, we can do as we like. And if communication was not something we believed to be important day-to-day then our motivation will fall and so will our effectiveness. Good communication is effortful and as other demands creep in it can fall down the priority list. We must all strive to ensure that we remain motivated to identify the task and communicate effectively to achieve it. You will discover, if you have not already, that the most powerful therapeutic tool you will ever have is your own personality, but you have to work at it.

The definition of effective medical communication

This may be the biggest obstacle of all. Communication in medicine is not the ability to have a good chat; it has to be related to diagnosis, treatment and outcome. The task of most medical encounters is to achieve a reasonable shared understanding with the patient of the phase of the medical cycle where both doctor and patient are. This is the problem with over-reliance on skills-based training. Communication skills are all very well but they can easily just become shallow tricks of the trade without remembering their purpose. The purpose, as we have pointed out in this little book, is to tap into our patient's health beliefs while performing our medical diagnostic and treatment manoeuvres and at the end of each interaction leave our patient as informed as their capacity will allow.

Some 20 years ago, as we have mentioned, Peter and others were involved in developing a competency-based examination for aspiring family doctors. They modelled this on an National Vocational Qualification (NVQ) model and adapted the seven communication tasks from Pendleton *et al.* (1984) (Peter is one of the authors.) The very first edition of this handbook was intended partly as a guide to this new examination. The examination was based on a driving test model, in that you the candidate had to demonstrate that you possessed that particular competence. Like the driving test some wishful thinking was associated, namely the hope that you would subsequently use this competence in your medical career, highlighting the big problem with competence: *it is not the same as performance in the workplace*. This particular examination involved submitting several candidate-selected recordings with real patients chosen to demonstrate the asked-for competencies. The examination lasted 10 years and its remains are clearly visible in the workplace-based communication assessment in general practice.

There is no doubt that clearly delineating the necessary components of competent consulting helps doctors to improve. We hope this little book helps you do just that, but defining and knowing the competencies is not the same as using them regularly; the question is not can you do it, but do you do it?

Reference

Pendleton D, Schofield T, Tate P, *et al. The Consultation: an approach to learning and teaching.* Oxford: Oxford University Press; 1984.

CHAPTER 13

Special situations and patients

Breaking bad news

This is not easy to do, and it can be such a daunting prospect that many doctors try all sorts of diversions and strategies to avoid doing it. 'Nurses are so much better at that sort of thing' is one of the excuses given. The reasons for this shying away from the task are usually emotional. Causing distress in another person causes distress in us. Therefore many of us do not perform very well in this crucial area of doctor–patient communication.

Common faults in breaking bad news

- Just not doing it, and hoping that someone else will pick up the pieces, such as the GP, another colleague, or one of the nursing staff. Common methods of doing this include avoiding the patient, never seeing them alone, or always being in a hurry. Trainees in hospital are exposed to this dilemma all the time. Virtually every encounter with an acutely unwell patient involves breaking bad news in some form and many prefer to gloss over it, dress it up or simply sidestep the issue entirely. This is largely out of fear and lack of experience. There is also a vague feeling that 'important' jobs such as this could be done better by someone else or that perhaps they are someone else's job.

- I'm sure the boss will be along later in the week. She'll explain everything.
- We just need to do a few more tests.

- Lying, or at best being economical with the truth.

> - We took the whole breast away and the affected glands. I'm sure we took it all away.
> - You will soon be better after the chemotherapy.
> - No, it's not too serious; we can cure it for you.

- Deliberately not picking up patient cues.

> Mrs Poole, aged 89, has metastatic breast cancer and has already been told there is no further treatment planned. She comes into the emergency department with severe shortness of breath. While the doctor takes a blood test, having taken a perfunctory clerking, she says: 'I know this is probably it, doctor. It's OK, I've had a good life.'
>
> Horrified, the doctor doesn't know what to say. The needle is still in her arm.
>
> Dr F eventually says: 'I'm sure it won't come to that. You're in good hands here,' and leaves hurriedly.

or

> Patient: I seem to be fading away, doctor.
> Dr: Really, how are you sleeping?
> Patient: The treatment isn't working, is it, doctor?
> Dr: Well, perhaps you are a little constipated.

- Going into undertaker mode, with excessive solemnity and an aura of deepening gloom. Lying is one thing, but excessive objectivity without mitigation is just as bad.
- Avoiding social and emotional issues. A study of oncologists in 1996 found that the doctors used closed questions and seldom gave the patients space to initiate any discussion. Although the patients must have been frightened, with all sorts of fears, only

1% of their talk was related to their concerns. To use a piece of jargon discussed earlier, the level of 'patient-centeredness' was very low. In this study patients were well informed about their diagnosis, prognosis and treatment options, but their emotional well-being was rarely probed. There were almost no social questions from the doctors, and the researchers found that the level of expressed empathy from the doctors was as low as 1%.

- Not recognising that emotion may block the patient's ability to take in much information.

Useful strategies to help you break bad news to patients

- Honesty is the best policy. Never tell patients anything that you know is not true. The truth will emerge over time, and the feelings of betrayal and of being misled will surface and sour your relationship both with your patient and with their family.
- Do not, however, tell the patient more than they want to know. This implies the need for a skilful manoeuvre to find out how much information they can cope with.
- Take great care with prognostications. *Never* give a specific time period – it will only come back to haunt you. You will almost certainly be wrong, and the effect on your patient will be depressing. Hope will ebb away and anxiety will increase as the stated time approaches. However, most patients do want some guidance on what the future holds for them.
- Do not remove all hope. Find some reason to be optimistic. The condition may be terminal, but you can encourage the patient to look forward to a particular event, such as a birth or celebration of an anniversary, or they may be hoping for a period of remission or for a peaceful, pain-free death.
- Remember the duty of confidentiality that is owed to your patient. This tends to go out of the window as soon as serious illness is suspected. Doctors have become used to ushering spouses into darkened corners and whispering terrible intimate details of their loved one's condition without a by-your-leave to the unfortunate sufferer. This has always been assumed to be for the patient's well-being. A study reported in the *British Medical Journal* in 1996 concluded that almost all patients, however ill, wanted to know their diagnosis, and most of them wanted to know about the prognosis, treatment options and side effects.

In the same issue, another study showed that patients rejected unconditional disclosure of information without their consent. They valued respect for their autonomy more highly than the medical beneficence, and considered that their own needs took priority over those of their family.

- Follow-up after giving bad news is especially important.

Useful skills to help you break bad news to patients

- Use your eliciting skills as described in Chapter 9.
- Ask yourself the question: 'How might this news affect this patient?' Think of the patient's family setting and their psychological make-up. Many patients are more worried about the effect of the bad news on others than they are about themselves.
- Consider the use of a tape recorder. This technique is now being used with increasing frequency in oncology departments. The evidence suggests that the patients and their relatives listen to the recordings on several occasions.
- Ask patients directly how much they know about the 'bad news'. For example, remember Mrs Arthur. Let us suppose that a thyroid scan has suggested a malignancy in one of the nodules, and a biopsy has confirmed this. She comes back to you for the report and your advice on further treatment. How do you proceed? Try the following type of approach:

Mrs Arthur: I have been so worried, doctor. What did the biopsy show?'

Doctor: Do you know why we did the biopsy?

Mrs Arthur: Yes, to see if it was cancer. Was it that, doctor?

Doctor: Yes, it was. I know that is bad news, but the outlook is not as bad as you think. Tell me what thyroid cancer means to you.

Mrs Arthur: Does this mean it will spread right through me? Will I die?

Doctor: No on both counts. We should be able to remove the gland and the cancer, and make sure it does not return by giving you some radiation treatment.

Mrs Arthur: That doesn't sound very nice – are you sure you can stop the cancer?

> Doctor: There is always a risk that we can't, but you would be very unlucky. The treatment I mentioned is very effective. Would you like to speak to someone more expert than me about it?
>
> Mrs Arthur: Well, not today, but I could I bring my husband along to see you and perhaps the other doctor you just mentioned?

- There is a lot more information you could give Mrs Arthur, and she may well want it, in time, but using the patient-centred approach as above enables the patient to take in only as much information with its unpleasant implications as they can cope with at one time.
- Be especially sensitive. Abrupt and brutal honesty, associated with authoritarian patient control, has no place in modern medicine. For example, consider the case of Mrs Arthur again. The following type of approach is not recommended:

> The test shows it's cancer, I'm afraid. We are bringing you in tomorrow morning to have the gland out. You can't hang around when cancer is about. OK?

- You must show consideration for your patient's feelings. Allow them time to think of questions and then you must answer them, and assure them of ongoing support. It is much better if bad news is given in the context of a continuing, supportive relationship. Do not give bad news and then make a run for it. Sit down with your patient and take your time. A pleasant, warm and safe setting is preferable. Try to ensure that there is someone else with the patient when you leave. You may need (with the patient's permission) to contact their partner or a close friend.
- When discussing the prognosis, remember that if your patient asks 'How long have I got?', they are already formulating an answer. You could say something like 'Well, I know you are poorly, but I think you have some time left, but how does it look to you?' Their answer may help you to deepen the discussion. What about the question 'Shall I ask my brother to come back from Australia?' I try answering this type of question with

another: 'Well, put yourself in their shoes. How would you feel if you were too late?'

- Learn to recognise and cope with *denial*. We all deal with devastating news in different ways. Many people cope by using varying degrees of denial. During your career you will experience situations where you have what you consider to be a sensitive, honest chat with a patient, containing a great deal of information, and then at the next consultation the patient will completely deny having had the conversation: 'They never told me anything at the hospital.'
- It is not a good strategy to break down denial too brutally. It is there for a purpose. Respect for the individual should extend to their defence mechanisms. This does not mean that we ourselves have to be a party to the denial and start encouraging unrealistic expectations. We must still reply honestly to any questions. It also means that we must pick up on rather obvious patient cues, such as 'The hospital doctor said it was just a little tumour. What a relief it isn't cancer, doctor.'
- Family denial or collusion is another problem more commonly encountered in general practice. Patients' capacity for denial is fascinating. Liz found working in a hospice as a trainee was illuminating. Even patients who had been told they had terminal cancer and were inpatients in a cancer hospice still cheerfully talked of holidays planned for the future and events they would never see. At this stage many declined help with making wills or planning funerals, causing much distress to family members. They would also decline to participate in shared decisions about end-of-life care. As the junior doctor on the ward it was tempting to run off to find a consultant each time this happened to break the news *again* rather than risk tearing down their defence mechanism herself. But it was important to resist this temptation and recognise that the duties of a doctor do not solely apply to seniors. Typically, a bit of time spent exploring the patient's beliefs and expectations helped them move to a more realistic place where they could address the future pragmatically. More often than not the patient was relieved themselves by achieving this degree of acceptance and open participation in end-of-life decisions.

It was also astonishing how few terminally ill people in the hospice had thought about, or had any opportunity to discuss, resuscitation or end-of-life care. This is done so poorly in many hospital wards probably due to a combination of lack of time and avoidance from juniors.

Don't tell him, doctor, it will kill him.

- This can lead to a tragic conspiracy of silence. The sufferer knows full well that their condition is terminal, but they cannot talk to their loved ones for fear of upsetting them. The loved ones in turn are so afraid of upsetting the sufferer in their last few weeks that nothing about the illness, about dying, about saying goodbye, etc., is discussed – to the detriment of all concerned. Partners collude because they love their other half and they don't want to hurt them – collusion is always a two-way process.
- Here we think there is a place for sensitive intervention by the doctor to try to break this pernicious circle. We believe firmly that our responsibility is to the patient, and that any responsibility to the family is secondary. In this type of situation we should tell the relatives that we would not impose the truth on the patient, but that if the patient asks we shall not lie. Often, with experience and tact, we can persuade all parties to talk reasonably openly about the future and help the patient towards a much more rewarding death, with a normal and not exaggerated grief to follow. This facilitation of family dynamics can be one of the more satisfying events in which we doctors can become involved.
- Use emotive words with care. Whatever the words 'cancer', 'tumour', 'growth', 'metastases', 'vegetative', 'malignant', 'thrombosis', etc., mean to you, it is certain that they do not mean the same thing to your patient. Check their understanding frequently, and remember that some people, cultures and societies have taboos relating to words like cancer. Be careful.
- Give your patient space to take it in. Pause, touch, empathise, commiserate, and use silence. Try to help to pick up the pieces. This can be emotionally painful for you, too.
- Remember that for the patient this is a momentous occasion. People recall the how, where and when very clearly, and you

– as the doctor – are wielding immense power. A woman of our acquaintance told me that when the young hospital doctor gave her better than expected news about her cancer, 'I was so pleased I could have married him.'

- Be prepared to spread the explanations over several consultations. It can help to ask the patient to write down questions as they come into their head and to bring them along to the next consultation.
- It is also true that what is bad news for one person may not be so for another. Peter was commiserating with an old patient of his about her dying husband when she exploded: 'Don't worry about me, doc. The old bugger has been driving me mental for years. The quicker he goes the better.'
- Just to recap, a paper published in the *British Medical Journal* (Kirk *et al.*, 2004) described a study from Canada and Australia of what patients receiving palliative care for cancer wanted to know. Six doctor attributes necessary for sensitive sharing of information were identified:
  ‣ playing it straight
  ‣ staying the course
  ‣ giving time
  ‣ showing that you care
  ‣ making it clear
  ‣ pacing the information.

Angry patients

This is another difficult emotional area, especially if the anger is directed towards you or one of your colleagues. Being ill can make people angry, so doctors are going to encounter a lot more than their fair share of this emotion. They may also be angry because we don't agree with them or won't do what they have demanded! There are many other reasons why patients get angry, including excessive waiting times and delayed appointments. Distress for another, often mixed with righteous indignation about the perceived medical failings, sometimes results in very intense and unpleasant encounters. There may be concerns that what the patient feels has not been taken seriously, disappointment at the lack of therapeutic success, and simple misunderstandings (especially when the patient expects one treatment but receives another, and the doctor has failed to explain the rationale). Guilt felt by patients or relatives that somehow they should have come sooner or cared for the patient better is a common reason for anger being directed at doctors. Anger is natural in grief and when adjusting to a serious diagnosis – the 'Why me?' effect. For most angry patients and relatives, anxiety is often the trigger.

Strategies for recognising and dealing with angry patients

- Remember that it is the patient/relative/carer who is angry, not you. This may be difficult, depending on your temperament. It is all too common for a simple misunderstanding to develop into a huge row, the worst place for this being the waiting room, where other patients can watch and take sides. Consider the environment. Notice how customer service people take angry complainants aside, away from everyone else. This is partly to avoid the spectacle and partly to reduce the stimulus around. Taking people to a quieter area reduces their arousal and also signifies you are concentrating on them. Obviously, this is more difficult if they are in your consulting room in primary care, but the sheer process of taking them through from the waiting room may help to begin this process.
- Do not leave the anger unexplored. Glowering at each other throughout the consultation is not effective and is bad for coronary arteries.
- Use your own feelings. If you are feeling angry, it is very likely that the patient is, too. Doctors feel anger if their competence is questioned or if they feel that their integrity is being challenged. After all, doctors are human, too, and a lack of appreciation from palpably ungrateful patients can make us cross, especially if we feel that we have made a special effort.
- Be patient – anger does not usually last for long.
- Always support your staff in the face of aggression that is really aimed at you. This is both a moral suggestion and a practical one. If you don't provide such support, before long you will not have any staff left.

Skills for defusing angry patients

- When you recognise anger, gentle confrontation may be helpful.

> - You seem to be cross about something.
> - Help, you do look upset.
> - Come on, get it off your chest; what is bothering you?
> - You were very angry with the nurse/receptionist. Why was that?

- In communication terms anger has a purpose – to gain the listener's (in this case the doctor's) complete attention. It is wise to let this happen.
- When you are listening, maintain non-threatening eye contact. Try not to raise your eyebrows, purse your lips or adopt an aggressive stance. When you speak, break off eye contact from time to time to demonstrate your wish to be conciliatory.
- Deal with the main issue first. Summarise the main points and then check them.
- Acknowledge the frailties and imperfections of medical diagnosis and treatment. Again honesty remains the best policy. A perceived delay in diagnosis or treatment is a common cause of patient anger. However, frankness about the nature of the delay will often diffuse this.
- Acknowledge your own lack of omnipotence, and watch the effects of your own guilt feelings. If you do not bring some of these feelings into the open, your relationship may be irrevocably harmed. Peter visited a little girl some time ago and thought that she had mild flu. A few hours later his partner admitted her with acute lobar pneumonia. The parents were angry about his perceived incompetence and told the partner so, and Peter was angry with himself and felt guilty for missing the diagnosis. He went to see the family, feeling rather ill at ease, after the little girl had been discharged, and expressed pleasure at her recovery and regrets about not diagnosing the pneumonia. The mother said:

> It was not your fault, doctor. You did examine her and you can't be right all the time. It did come on pretty quickly.

And the family continued to be his patients.

Another effective technique for dealing with angry people involves matching their communication style. The idea is that you can help to de-escalate the situation by matching them closely and then, once you are in control, shifting and bringing them with you. Try to subtly match their position (without obviously mimicking them which will probably annoy them further). If they are standing up and you are sitting down there is an imbalance. You will feel more vulnerable and they will feel more powerful. Stand up yourself and then perhaps if things are going well try sitting down and see if they follow suit. If not, stand up again. Try to match their demeanour. Obviously, avoid shouting yourself, but if they are talking loudly and you try to respond in a timid meek voice there is an imbalance. Raise your voice a bit until you are both on a level then try to bring theirs down with you.

Validation is usually key. Tempting as it is to jump in with defences and refutations, particularly when we are being attacked personally, it is much better to listen for a couple of minutes with perhaps 'I can see how difficult that must have been for you' and 'I am sure if I was in your position I would feel angry, too'. It is surprising how effective this can be.

The reason for anger will dictate the way it is managed. Someone who is angry at a missed diagnosis will need time to vent, an apology if warranted and then careful exploration of their understanding and next steps. Someone who is angrily demanding a prescription for methadone will need a different approach involving careful negotiation and an understanding that a shared decision may not be reached in this instance. When negotiating in this instance be clear with the patient what you can and can't do for them and your bottom line. Use your active listening to the maximum – summarise, clarify, reframe and check. Try to empathise even when this may be difficult. Stay credible and honest, and listen to their perspective. If necessary ask for time to think. Try not to be punitive, make assumptions or be intimidated into making unwise or hasty decisions.

Other strategies to consider when dealing with angry people, including during a difficult phone call, are the following.

- Apologise sincerely (but don't accept the blame unless it really is your fault).
- Be diplomatic, appear to be interested in resolving the issue.

- Be professional at all times, don't rise to the bait or become emotional.
- Don't get defensive or into an argument.
- Allow them to vent (just listen).
- Use empathy – say you can see why there are upset.
- Thank them for their response: 'Thanks for being so honest/ flagging the problem to me'.
- Watch out for escalation – change in speed or tone of voice, going quiet.
- Try to offer solutions if appropriate.
- Be aware how you come across. Impressions matter. Try to convey enthusiasm, a genuine desire to help and cheerfulness, where appropriate.
- Summarise and check you have understood the information.
- Don't hang up if on the phone.
- Make sure you get their name and contact details if you don't have these already.
- Finish off positively, ideally by summarising the action plan.
- Some people feel the anonymity of the phone means they can be as rude as they like as they aren't face to face with a human. Try to counter this by introducing a human element like mentioning your kids or saying something like 'I am not personally responsible for this situation but I will help to sort it out with you'.
- Use repetition. Stick to your guns.
- Make good notes afterwards. Take excellent notes from any incident involving an angry person to ensure you have an accurate record of what was said by you both.
- Someone who is so angry they are ranting might need quite an assertive approach: 'I really want to help sort this out, but I need you to tell me what exactly has been happening – can you talk me through it from the beginning?'
- Above all, *never* say 'Calm down' to an angry person!
- When there seems to be a real threat of physical violence, and you have made every effort to defuse the situation, avoid physical confrontation. If possible, move away and get help. If you have a panic button, press it.

The somatising patient

Another common difficulty is the patient who attends repeatedly with physical illness that is unclassifiable by an increasingly investigative doctor. The unexplained breathlessness, the fleeting chest pains, the weird pins and needles – all possible precursors of nasty diseases. However, we have to remember that common things are common, most illnesses are not serious and most symptoms are not disease. They are problems of living turned into symptoms by anxious people and turned into disease by biologically trained doctors. Patients who are prone to turning inner anxieties into symptoms are called somatisers. Doctors who turn such symptoms into disease have been called medicalisers. As we mentioned in Chapter 5, a medicalising doctor and a somatising patient are a bad combination.

These are the patients we find especially difficult; the ones who ask 'What are you going to do about my . . .?' They get labelled 'heartsink' patients in general practice, and in hospital they are very quickly 'turfed' from the senior staff to their junior colleagues. The really chronic somatiser does not have their notes inspected – they have them weighed. This sad, irritating and enormously time-consuming state of affairs is the result of a long process of medicalisation by doctors and the health industry, including alternative medicine, of essentially nervous and functional complaints made by introspective individuals. These people often have a 'powerful other' locus of control, although fussy internal controllers can get doctors down, too. Curiously, fatalists do not commonly produce such negative emotions.

The problem with doctors in this context is that if patients keep pushing we will eventually do something. This could be a test, which will lead to a procedure, which can lead to an operation, which can lead to a complication, which in turn will reinforce the patient's inappropriate health-seeking behaviour.

> See, I was ill, doctor. I am a lot better after my triple artery graft. Now about these headaches . . .

Most experienced doctors know personally a group of patients who have had coronary artery surgery not because their arteries were in any worse shape than most, but because they persistently kept presenting different symptoms to different doctors. This led to tests being performed that were equivocal, as tests tend to be, but the pressure for something to be done meant that in the end something was done. These patients had thick sets of notes before and even thicker ones afterwards. So what can we doctors do about this?

Strategies for decreasing our patients' tendency to become somatically fixated and medically dependent

- Use the communication methods described earlier in this book, with particular emphasis on achieving a shared understanding and shared management plan. Patients should be encouraged to take some responsibility for their own health.
- Use the traditional disease-based medical model with care. Although we all need to be good diagnosticians, good efficient clinical practice demands balances – most headaches do not warrant MRI scans. Investigation on demand is bad medicine, and treatment on demand may be worse. We must not create disease where only poor individual coping mechanisms are the problem. This can mean trying to change the patient's purely biomechanical view of illness. Psychologists call this the defusion of the organic versus the functional, and they use strategies to help patients to 'reattribute' their explanations for ill health. These strategies include emphasising the role of anxiety in muscular tension, pain and hyperventilation, the effect of depression on pain thresholds, and the vicious circle of pain and psychological distress.
- Remember ICE! A study reported in the *British Journal of General Practice* (Nijrolder *et al.*, 2009) showed that the strongest predictor of poor outcome in patients presenting with fatigue was their expectation of chronicity.
- Be on your guard against behaviour that can come across as manipulative. Often individuals are labelled as 'manipulative' unfairly when they are simply acting in a way consistent with their own concerns and expectations in the face of resistance and lack of sympathy from health professionals! It is essential to spot this process and attempt to address it directly rather than simply say it's the patient's problem.
- Family doctors must think hard about referral. Only when all reasonable avenues and likely diagnoses have been refuted should a referral to outpatients be made. We still believe that one of the

GP's primary duties is to protect his or her patients from hospital medicine. Hospital medicine is almost exclusively disease-based; patients must be diagnosed thoroughly and possible causes ruled out. Once an anxious, introspective patient gets to outpatients the die is cast – investigation is coming and all that that might entail. The fixation with the symptom will be intensified and the vicious self-reinforcing loop encouraged. Referrals should only be made for the following reasons:

- for *diagnostic reasons* (i.e. the further testing of a specific hypothesis, the resources for which you do not possess)
- for *therapeutic purposes* (if you do not want or are unable to treat a certain condition)
- for *reassurance*. This is the really tricky one. Even if there is no traditional disease, the modern hospital's ability to dig up some minor disorder which is essentially irrelevant, and to overtreat it, is formidable. This can of course lead to further referral. There is also the danger that, not unreasonably, you or your chief may ask the patient to return on the grounds that although you have drawn a blank, you may have overlooked something. Both of these situations will probably lead the patient to conclude that they were right, and that there is something wrong with their health. For example, the 42-year-old woman patient with atypical chest pain who insisted on referral has a non-specific minor anomaly in a couple of leads of the ECG. This leads to echocardiography which is essentially OK, and to a treadmill test which is also essentially OK, but with a performance nearer the bottom end of the normal range than the top. This leads to a full catheterisation, which is essentially normal, but no one's arteries are entirely normal, and the patient overhears your discussion of her essentially normal variants with rising anxiety. Her consequent release of catecholamines and irritation of previously untouched places by the catheter produce a minor arrhythmia that you need to respond to quickly and (in her eyes) dramatically. Her worst fears are confirmed and the seeds of cardiac crippledom are well and truly sown.

- The reasons for referral should be explicit, and the doctor who accepts the referral should whenever possible keep within the mandate of the referral letter.

- Try to keep the numbers of doctors involved with a particular patient to a minimum. The more doctors there are involved, the more somatisation there will be.
- Keep good records. You need to let partners and other doctors know what your plans are, whether you fear a somatising process is happening to the patient, and your strategies for preventing further harm.
- Communicate with your colleagues about patients you suspect of undue somatisation leading to 'doctor shopping' (i.e. consulting every doctor in the practice in turn for another opinion, or swapping specialists frequently).
- Write explicit and detailed referral letters. These should contain biographical details, clinical and physical symptoms and signs, the course of the complaint, your own hypotheses, the previous history, important psychosocial background information, and the beliefs and wishes of the patient. There should also be a clear statement of what you are asking of your colleague, and what you wish to happen after your colleague has seen the patient.
- Use patient diaries and other methods of self-recording to try to produce more insight and linkage between events and symptoms.

Skills for preventing and dealing with somatisation

- Use the concepts of transactional analysis. You are trying to achieve an adult–adult relationship, not a parent–child relationship. Read Eric Berne's *Games People Play* (1964).
- Discuss your perceptions of your patient's illness behaviour.

- You have been coming to see me a lot recently, and I never seem to find much wrong. What do you expect of me?
- It is a year since your heart attack and you still seem to be leaving everything to your wife to do. It is as if you do not want to get better.

- Discuss the patient's methods of denial and avoidance.

> - Every time I ask you if anything is troubling you, you say to me 'Nobody has a perfect life' and leave it at that, but you keep coming to me with problems that I can't really help you with. You will have to help me more before I can help you.
> - I know you have not been well in the last year. Today it is your sinuses, last time it was your tummy pain and before that your headaches. Do you think there is something worrying you underneath all this?
> - You are trying to blame everything on a virus, but I think you are not facing the real problem of your anxiety.

- Try to verbalise your patient's anxiety.

> - You are afraid it is something serious, aren't you?
> - You seem very tense. Are you frightened of something?
> - If you go on worrying about yourself you are going to get into a vicious circle, don't you think?
> - You have been panicking a bit recently, but nothing serious has developed. Can you get any comfort from that?

- Use the presenting signals from the minimal cues.

> - You seem much more anxious than normal.
> - It looks to me that something is really troubling you.

- Describe to the patient the way in which they are trying to influence you.

- I know you would like me to send you to see a specialist, but I do not think that is necessary. I am not sure what to do next.
- I think you want me to give you a pill and then expect all your troubles will be over, but I don't think it is as easy as that.
- The way you are behaving gives me the feeling you are saying, 'Please help me. I don't know which way to turn.' Am I right?

- Discuss and use your own feelings.

- Honestly, I have tried everything and I don't know where to go from here. Have you any suggestions?
- I am sorry, but you have made me feel inadequate and unable to help you. Can you help me to help you?

- Clarify the patient's complaint(s), to give them more insight.

I think your headache is caused by the muscles in the neck going into spasm. This is why painkillers don't work very well – they don't relieve the spasm. It is probably your worrying about your mum that caused the muscle spasm in the first place.

- Try to avoid giving too much advice to these patients. Any advice should be specific (i.e. to give a new approach to the problem), and it should be realistically tailored to the individual patient.
- Encourage the patient's internal search, and encourage them to find their own solutions and alternative strategies.

Motivational interviewing approaches can also work here. This is a patient-centred approach designed to help facilitate a change in health-related behaviour. A meta-analysis study found this approach was much more effective than simple advice giving (Rubak *et al.*, 2005).

Useful questions here are:

- What would you most like to talk about?
- How important is it to change . . .?
- How might things be different if . . .?
- How confident do you feel about changing . . .?

Helping people quantify and rate things can also help them seem more manageable for you both. Someone who experiences chronic pain described as 'terrible' which dominates their life may, on further exploration, actually have times in the day where the pain is only 5/10 and they can get out to walk the dog. Perhaps the worst time is the evening when they are tired and the pain goes up to 9/10 and this could be the area for your initial focus. Pain teams often have no better treatments than anyone else but are experts in this approach and see results.

Goal setting

In the face of seemingly insurmountable problems, helping the patient to set more manageable goals can be useful.

Rather than:

> 'I'm just tired and achy all the time doctor. I don't know what to do any more.'
>
> 'Well, Mrs Jones we have talked about this before. There is really nothing I can do to help with this. I suggested stopping smoking and going to bed earlier and I'm not sure what else to say.'

Try:

> 'I see this is still a real problem for you. It must be getting you down. Shall we focus on the tiredness today and look at that a bit more? When is it worse for you? What does it stop you doing?'
>
> 'It's worse in the morning, which is a pain because I used to enjoy taking the grandchildren to school.'
>
> 'So if you were able to start doing that again this would be a step forward?'

'Well, yes. That would actually make me feel much better.'
'So how about we look at ways to improve things in the morning to see if we can help you take the kids to school again?'

- Don't let such patients get you down.

Remember that many patients with somatising disorders are depressed as well as anxious.

Counselling skills

Counselling is a difficult area for the untrained doctor. There is no agreement on what counselling methodologies should be adopted, how effective the various strategies are and how to find the time in the first place. In the Google dictionary counselling is defined as something that provides direction or advice as to a decision or course of action. This is a robustly simple description that gives us some hope that most of our day-to-day work in the surgery could be described as counselling.

Any effective doctor–patient interaction should contain large amounts of the first accepted counselling skill, active listening. This skill in enhanced by the seeking out of belief systems highlighted by the listening and then utilising the higher level skill of synthesising this information into a narrative that can be understood. This information needs to be stored until the time comes in the consultation to respond to the problem or scenario your patient has presented. Almost all significant problems brought to doctors require a professional response with advice on possible courses of action and allowing the element of informed choice.

The professional counsellors will belong to one or other of three schools of thought: psychodynamic; humanistic; behavioural and cognitive. The first is essentially Freudian and unless you are that way inclined best avoided. Humanistic counselling is most commonly called Rogerian, though Maslow and his hierarchy of needs are a central tenet of this school of thought. Freud is still lurking in the background, and the actual skills used include active listening but almost no advice giving. The patient is enabled to see what they need to do by insight into their own condition from their own narrative, the aim being Maslow's pinnacle of human needs, self-actualisation. This type of counselling may suit some doctors, but it is time-consuming, requires a period of training and needs constant support.

The most popular form of counselling over the last decade is based on cognitive psychology and behaviourism and is labelled cognitive behavioural therapy (CBT). It is based on the attractively obvious theory that how we think (cognition), how we feel (emotion), and how we act (behaviour) are related and interact in complex ways.

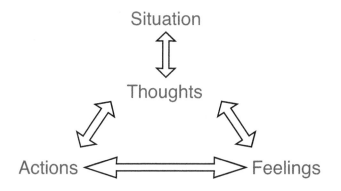

FIGURE 13.1 Interaction between cognition, emotion and behaviour

The great attraction of CBT to most doctors is the lack of mysticism, combined with a logical approach and the relative absence of psychoanalytical theory. In fact, it can be traced to Pavlov and his dogs and Skinner and his pigeons. As ever, the evidence base can be argued with, but it certainly appears to be the most scientifically supported method of talking therapy. This is, however, not a routine tool for most patient encounters; depending on the problem and the patient this form of counselling usually needs a limited number of, but several, sessions and does require expertise, time set aside and regular practice.

The underlying CBT concept of the patient being helped to help themselves by recognising and changing unhelpful thought patterns does lend itself to self-help programmes. There are currently two such available to NHS patients, Fear Fighter (www.fearfighter.com) is for people with phobias or panic attacks; Beating the Blues (www.beating theblues.co.uk) is for people with mild to moderate depression.

One of the main problems with the notion of 'counselling' is the perception induced by many sources including the media that it is a panacea for all experienced traumas and a necessary requirement in any form of shock and bereavement. It is also an unregulated growth industry with many substandard practitioners. The ridiculous situation has arisen over recent years of some doctors spending significant time counselling patients against 'counselling' or, worse, handing patients over to therapists, whose beliefs are usually unknown to them, as a way of washing their own hands of the problem.

References

Berne E. *Games People Play: the basic handbook of transactional analysis.* New York: Ballantine Books; 1964.

Kirk P, Kirk I, Kristjanson LJ. What do patients receiving palliative care for cancer and their families want to be told? A Canadian and Australian qualitative study. *BMJ.* 2004; **328**: 1343.

Nijrolder I, van der Windt D, van der Horst H. Prediction of outcome in patients presenting with fatigue in primary care. *Br J Gen Pract.* 2009; 59(561): e101–9.

Rubak S, Sandbaek A, Lauritzen T, *et al.* Motivational interviewing: a systematic review and meta-analysis. *Br J Gen Pract.* 2005; 55(513): 305–12.

CHAPTER 14

Summary

'The good physician treats the disease; the great physician treats the patient who has the disease.'
'It is much more important to know what sort of a patient has a disease than what sort of a disease a patient has.'
'Look wise, say nothing, and grunt. Speech was given to conceal thought.'
'Medicine is a science of uncertainty and an art of probability.'

a few Oslerisms

We wonder what you have learned from this book. The message we hope you will take away is that effective communication can be learned. That it is not just God-given and incapable of improvement. We can all do it better, but we have to believe that the effort is worthwhile and that the goal is an important one.

Let us summarise some of the very important messages, firstly about patients.

What doctors should know about patients

In hospital

The patient is more frightened than you are. They think that their condition is more serious than you do. Most of them want to be involved in their own treatment, and they want to understand what is going to happen to them.

They have not come to you about liver or thyroid disease. They have come because of their beliefs about, their expectations of and the effects of their perceived change in health. Remember, whenever possible, to try to put yourself in their shoes.

Your patient is probably afraid of you. They will tend to be passive and not say very much. This does not mean that they do not want to know.

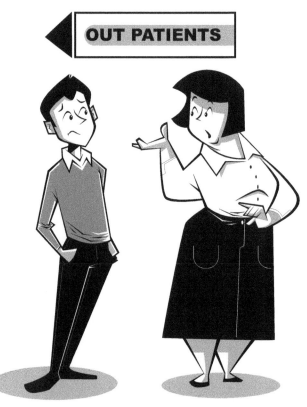

*"EEH, I WAS SO POORLY I DIDN'T EVEN
WANT TO TALK ABOUT IT"*

Patients are just people like you. They deserve respect, they need to be informed and they need to consent. However, people are all different, they respond to a change in health in different ways, and they need individual, personalised plans.

People can easily have inappropriate and unhelpful illness behaviour reinforced by poorly thought out and unexplained investigation and treatment. Patients will follow surprisingly little of your advice unless you really make an effort.

But they trust you, they really do.

In general practice

People want to make sense of any perceived change in their health. You may be the first person to whom they tell that particular story, and it may not make much sense if it is squeezed into the 'medical model'.

People come to you for guidance, advice and treatment. Reasonable health promotion is OK, but be careful not to step over the line into overzealous lifestyle advice.

People are less informed than you think. Many procedures and screening programmes require much more sharing of understanding.

What doctors should know about communication

Oscar Wilde said of England and America that we were divided by a common language. The same could be said of doctors and patients. Most patients do not know the difference between a virus, a bacterium and an amoeba – they are all bugs. Most GPs use the virus versus bacteria issue to bolster their arguments about antibiotic prescribing. How many patients are using the same frame of reference? Peter Havelock, a GP friend, told of the time he reviewed a recorded consultation with the patient, an elderly man. They watched it together, and at the end the old man made the following comments:

> Patient: Yes, doc. I thought that were good, but I was just a bit unhappy about one thing. You said you were going to give me antibiotics and then at the end you didn't.
> Doctor: But I gave you penicillin.
> Patient: Oh, I didn't realise thems were antibiotics.

Patients have clear expectations of what will happen in conversations with doctors. A local radio show held a competition for the event you would most like to happen but which would be most unlikely to happen to you. One of the winners was 'going to your doctor with a sore throat and getting antibiotics without an argument about viruses'. The potential for misunderstandings between doctors and patients is unlimited.

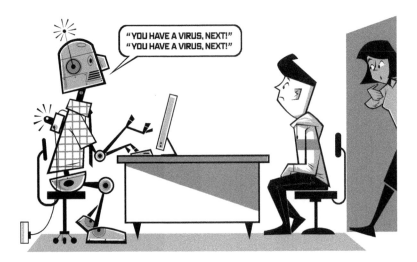

Out of the mass of research work on communication with patients, the following stark truths emerge.

- The amount of explanation that a patient receives is directly related to their intelligence as perceived by the doctor.
- The lower the patient's social class, the less explanation is offered. Yet all patients from the highest to the lowest and the brightest to the more intellectually challenged want as much information as they can assimilate, and in a form that they can understand. This is a very big challenge to our profession.
- Patients' and doctors' perceptions of patients' problems differ from those expressed both before and after their consultations. Their perceptions about the consultation itself also differ.
- Asking questions only gets you answers. This is one of the problems with traditional history taking – a method of putting communication into a straitjacket in order to maximise pattern recognition.
- Doctors are likely to consistently overestimate their patients' understanding. Written information, pamphlets and leaflets are useful but poorly understood by the majority of the population. Other problems with written material include it not being noticed, not being read and not being remembered.
- Doctors rarely talk to patients about the consequences of their illnesses. We do usually explain a little, but we rarely share what our patients think, and we also rarely check whether our patients

understand. Sharing any type of management is still unusual. Our consultations are very one-sided.

- To communicate effectively you must search for your patient's agenda and reconcile this with your own agenda. This is a skilful process, and the outcome should be a shared understanding and a shared management plan.

Interaction with a patient: summary

Let us now summarise again what you should seek to achieve in an interaction with a patient, in hospital or in general practice.

1 Discover the reason(s) why your patient has come to see you

To achieve this you will need to do the following.

- Try to understand your patient. To do this you will need to:
  - listen to them
  - pick up cues
  - obtain and use relevant social and occupational information
  - explore their health understanding
  - enquire about problems other than the presenting one.
- Try to understand the problem(s). To do this you will need to:
  - obtain additional information about critical symptoms and details of the medical history
  - assess your patient's condition by examination if appropriate
  - make a working diagnosis
  - assess the severity of the presenting problem.

2 Share understanding

To achieve this you will need to do the following.

- Share your findings with the patient.
- Tailor the explanation to the needs of the patient.
- Ensure that the explanation is understood and accepted by the patient.

3 Share decisions and responsibility

To achieve this you will need to do the following.

- Together with the patient, choose an appropriate form of management.
- Involve your patient in the management plan to the appropriate extent.

- Try to achieve a shared management plan.
- Ensure that the patient understands the plan.

4 Make effective use of the interaction
To achieve this you will need to do the following.
- Make efficient use of resources, including:
  - effective use of time
  - appropriate investigations
  - appropriate referral
  - appropriate concordant prescribing.
- Establish and maintain an effective relationship with your patient.
- Give opportunistic health advice where appropriate.
- Safety net effectively.

If you practise the completion of the above tasks, hone your present skills and learn some new ones as necessary, you will become a better doctor than you are now. Your patients should be happier and healthier, too.

Good communicating.

Appendix

Suggested reading

Since the early editions of this book were published, the concept of a reading list has been fundamentally changed by the Internet. Most articles now have electronically linked references, so there is no longer a need for a detailed list. What follows is a list of some of our favourite books and just a few modern review articles (from which further references can be obtained).

Essential books

Berne E. *Games People Play: the basic handbook of transactional analysis*. New York: Ballantine Books; 1964.

Kahneman D. *Thinking, Fast and Slow*. New York: Farrar, Straus and Giroux; 2011.

Neighbour R. *The Inner Consultation*. 2nd ed. Oxford: Radcliffe Publishing; 2005.

Pendleton D, Schofield T, Tate P, *et al. The New Consultation: developing doctor–patient communication*. Oxford: Oxford University Press; 2003.

Shem S. *The House of God*. New York: Dell Publishing; 1978.

Good value

Balint M. *The Doctor, His Patient and the Illness*. London: Tavistock Publications; 1957.

Byrne PS, Long BEL. *Doctors Talking to Patients: a study of the verbal behaviours of doctors in the consultation*. London: Her Majesty's Stationery Office; 1976.

Downie R, Macnaughton J. *Clinical Judgement: evidence in practice*. Oxford: Oxford University Press; 2000.

Drucquer M, Hutchinson S. *The Consultation Toolkit*. London: Reed Healthcare Publishing; 2000.

Edwards AGK, Elwyn G, editors. *Evidence-Based Patient Choice: inevitable or impossible?* Oxford: Oxford University Press; 2001.

Helman C. *Suburban Shaman: tales from medicine's front line.* London: Hammersmith Press; 2006.

Misselbrook D. *Thinking about Patients.* Newbury: Petroc Press; 2001.

Pendleton P, Hasler J, editors. *Doctor–Patient Communication.* London: Academic Press; 1983.

Pendleton D, Schofield T, Tate P, *et al. The Consultation: an approach to learning and teaching.* Oxford: Oxford University Press; 1984.

Salinsky J, Sackin P. *What Are You Feeling, Doctor? Identifying and avoiding defensive patterns in the consultation.* Oxford: Radcliffe Medical Press; 2000.

Silverman J, Kurtz S, Draper J. *Skills for Communicating with Patients.* 3rd ed. London: Radcliffe Publishing; 2013.

Skrabanek P. *The Death of Humane Medicine.* London: The Social Affairs Unit; 1994.

Stewart M, Brown JB, Weston WW, *et al. Patient-Centered Medicine: transforming the clinical method.* 3rd ed. London: Radcliffe Publishing; 2014.

Tuckett D, Boulton M, Olson C *et al. Meetings between Experts.* London: Tavistock Publications; 1985.

Relevant *British Medical Journal* issues

Communicating risks: illusion or truth? *BMJ.* 2003; **327**(7417).

Embracing patient partnership. *BMJ.* 1999; **319**(7212).

From compliance to concordance. *BMJ.* 2003; **327**(7419).

Too much medicine. *BMJ.* 2002; **342**(7342).

Recent articles on communication

Berwick D. The epitaph of profession. *Br J Gen Pract.* 2009; **59**: 128–31.

Elwyn G, Edwards A, Hood K *et al.* and the Study Steering Group. Achieving involvement: process outcomes from a cluster randomized trial of shared decision-making skill development and use of risk communication aids in general practice. *Fam Pract.* 2004; **21**: 337–46.

Griffin SJ, Kinmonth A-L, Veltman MWM *et al.* Effect on health-related outcomes of interventions to alter the interaction between patients and practitioners: a systematic review of trials. *Ann Fam Med.* 2004; **2**: 595–608.

Howie J, Heaney D, Maxwell M. Quality, core values and the general practice consultation: issues of definition, measurement and delivery. *Fam Pract.* 2004; **21**: 458–68.

Kidd J, Patel V, Peile E *et al.* Clinical and communication skills. *BMJ.* 2005; **330**: 374–5.

Kirk P, Kirk I, Kristjanson LJ. What do patients receiving palliative care for cancer and their families want to be told? A Canadian and Australian qualitative study. *BMJ*. 2004; **328**: 1343.

Little P, Everitt H, Williamson I *et al*. Observational study of effect of patient centredness and positive approach on outcomes of general practice consultations. *BMJ*. 2001; **322**: 908–11.

Loxterkamp D. Why rivers run: on the headwaters of family medicine. *BMJ*. 2008; **337**: a2575.

Matthys J, Elwyn G, Van Nuland M *et al*. Patients' ideas, concerns and expectations (ICE) in general practice: impact on prescribing. *Br J Gen Pract*. 2009; **59**: 29–36.

Ridd M, Shaw A, Lewis G *et al*. The patient–doctor relationship: a synthesis of the qualitative literature on patients' perspectives. *Br J Gen Pract*. 2009; **59**: 268–75.

Roberts J. Describing the road to death. *BMJ*. 2005; **331**: E364–5.

Stewart M. Reflections on the doctor–patient relationship: from evidence and experience. *Br J Gen Pract*. 2005; **55**: 793–801.

Other references

Austoker J. Gaining informed consent for screening is difficult – but many misconceptions need to be undone. *BMJ*. 1999; **319**: 722–3.

Barry CA, Bradley CP, Britten N *et al*. Patients' unvoiced agendas in general practice consultations: qualitative study. *BMJ*. 2000; **320**: 1246–50.

Baum M. Harms from breast cancer screening outweigh benefits if death by treatment included. *BMJ*. 2013; **346**: f385.

Blackburn DF, Swidrovich J, Lemstra M. Non-adherence in type 2 diabetes: practical considerations for interpreting the literature. *Patient Prefer Adherence*. 2013; **7**: 183–9.

Brito JP, Morris JC, Montori VM. Thyroid cancer: zealous imaging has increased detection and treatment of low risk tumours. *BMJ*. 2013; **347**: f4706.

Butler CC, Pill R, Stott NC. Qualitative study of patients' perceptions of doctors' advice to quit smoking: implications for opportunistic health promotion. *BMJ*. 1998; **316**(7148): 1878–81.

Cals JW, Butler CC, Hopstaken RM *et al*. Effect of point of care testing for C reactive protein and training in communication skills on antibiotic use in lower respiratory tract infections: cluster randomised trial. *BMJ*. 2009; **338**: b1374.

Department of Health. *Good Practice in Consent Implementation Guide*. Available online at: www.health.wa.gov.au/mhareview/resources/documents/UK_DOH_implementation_guide.pdf

Department of Health. *NHS Constitution*. London: Department of Health; 2013.

Fallowfield LJ, Hall A, Maguire GP, *et al.* Psychological outcomes of different treatment policies in women with early breast cancer outside a clinical trial. *BMJ.* 1990; **301**: 575–80.

Fowler FJ Jr, Gerstein BS, Barry MJ. How patient centered are medical decisions? Results of a national survey. *BMJ.* **173**(13): 1215–21.

Freeman GK, Horder JP, Howie JGR *et al.* Evolving general practice consultation in Britain: issues of length and context. *BMJ.* 2002; **324**(7342): 880–2.

General Medical Council. *Duties of a Doctor.* London: General Medical Council; 2000.

General Medical Council. *Seeking Patients' Consent: the ethical considerations.* London: General Medical Council; 1998.

Gigerenzer GW, Gaissmaier W, Kurz-Milcke E, *et al.* Helping doctors and patients make sense of health statistics. *Psychol Sci Public Interest.* 2008; **8**(2): 53–96.

Greenfield S, Kaplan S, Ware JE Jr. Expanding patient involvement in care: effects on patient outcomes. *Ann Intern Med.* 1985; **102**(4): 520–8.

Heath I. William Pickles Lecture 1999: 'Uncertain clarity': contradiction, meaning, and hope. *Br J Gen Pract.* 1999; **49**(445): 651–7.

Horder JP, Byrne PS, Freeling P, *et al. The Future General Practitioner: learning and teaching.* London: The Royal College of General Practitioners; 1972.

Horne R. Compliance, adherence, and concordance: implications for asthma treatment. *Chest.* 2006; **130**(1 Suppl): S65–72.

Horne R, Weinman J, Barber N, *et al. Concordance, adherence and compliance in medicine taking.* 2005. Available at: www.nets.nihr.ac.uk/__data/assets/pdf_file/0009/64494/FR-08-1412-076.pdf

Illich I. *Medical Nemesis.* London: Marion Boyars; 1975.

Illman J, Kirkness B, Association of British Pharmaceutical Industry. *The Expert Patient.* London: Association of the British Pharmaceutical Association; 2000.

Jørgensen KJ, Gøtzsche PC. Overdiagnosis in publicly organised mammography screening programmes: systematic review of incidence trends. *BMJ.* 2009; **339**: b2587.

McCarthy M. Harms of PSA screening outweigh benefits for most men, says American College of Physicians. *BMJ.* 2013; **346**: f2232.

McKinstry B. Do patients wish to be involved in decision making in the consultation? A cross sectional survey with video vignettes. *BMJ.* 2000; **321**(7265): 867–71.

McKinstry B, Watson P, Pinnock H, *et al.* Telephone consulting in primary care: a triangulated qualitative study of patients and providers. *Br J Gen Pract.* 2009; **59**: 202–18.

Mjaaland TA, Finset A, Jensen BF, *et al.* Physicians' responses to patients' expressions of negative emotions in hospital consultations: a video-based observational study. *Patient Educ Couns.* 2011; **84**(3): 332–7.

Mulley AG, Trimble C, Elwyn G. Stop the silent misdiagnosis: patients' preferences matter. *BMJ*. 2012; **345**: e6572.

Nijrolder I, van der Windt D, van der Horst H. Prediction of outcome in patients presenting with fatigue in primary care. *Br J Gen Pract*. 2009; **59**(561): e101–9.

Prochaska JO, DiClemente CC. Stages and processes of self-change in smoking: toward an integrative model of change. *J Consul Clin Psychol*. 1983; **51**(3): 390–5.

Rubak S, Sandbaek A, Lauritzen T, *et al*. Motivational interviewing: a systematic review and meta-analysis. *Br J Gen Pract*. 2005; **55**(513): 305–12.

Shelford G. Risks, statistics, and the individual. *BMJ*. 2003; **327**: 757.

Shepherd HL, Barratt A, Trevena LJ *et al*. Three questions that patients can ask to improve the quality of information physicians give about treatment options: a cross-over trial. *Patient Educ Couns*. 2011; **84**(3): 379–85.

Smith SK, Trevena L, Simpson JM *et al*. A decision aid to support informed choices about bowel cancer screening among adults with low education: randomised controlled trial. *BMJ*. 2010; **341**: c5370.

Stimson GV, Webb B. *Going to See the Doctor*. London: Routledge & Keegan Paul; 1975.

Tongue JR, Epps HR, Forese LL. Communication skills for patient-centered care: research-based, easily learned techniques for medical interviews that benefit orthopaedic surgeons and their patients. *J Bone Joint Surg Am*. 2005; **87**: 652–8.

Watson C. The P value of empathy. *BMJ*. 2005; **330**(7482): 101.

Index

Note: entries in **bold** refer to figures and tables.

CPD with Radcliffe

You can now use a selection of our books to achieve CPD (Continuing Professional Development) points through directed reading.

We provide a free online form and downloadable certificate for your appraisal portfolio. Look for the CPD logo and register with us at: www.radcliffehealth.com/cpd

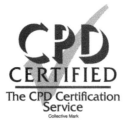

CPD CERTIFIED
The CPD Certification
Service
Collective Mark